American Medicine

American Medicine: The Quest for Competence

Mary-Jo DelVecchio Good

UNIVERSITY OF CALIFORNIA PRESS

Berkeley / Los Angeles / London

University of California Press
Berkeley and Los Angeles, California

University of California Press
London, England

Library of Congress Cataloging-in-Publication Data
Good, Mary-Jo DelVecchio.
    American medicine: The quest for competence / Mary-Jo
DelVecchio Good.
      p.   cm.
    Includes bibliographical references and index.
    ISBN 0–520–08896–4 (cloth: alk. paper)
    1. Clinical competence.   2. Medical care—United States—
Evaluation.   I. Title.
    [DNLM: 1. Clinical Competence.   2. Physicians.
3. Professional Autonomy.   4. Education, Medical—United
States.   W 21 G646a 1995]
RA399.A3G66   1995
362.1'0973—dc20
DNLM/DLC   94–36162
for Library of Congress   CIP

Printed in the United States of America

1 2 3 4 5 6 7 8 9

For my parents
Frank and Filomena DelVecchio

What do we care about? "What do we care about?" is the hardest question in all of medicine.

—A newly graduated physician

Contents

Acknowledgments

Three research studies form the ethnographic heart of this book. The study of rural medicine in California was partially funded by two research grants from the National Institute of Mental Health, which were flexible enough to incorporate a more general ethnography of medical practice into a clinical epidemiology project on mental health and primary care. The project on the New Pathway and innovation in medical education at Harvard Medical School was supported by the medical school, without paradigm or political constraints, through a grant from the Henry J. Kaiser Family Foundation. The Cummings Foundation, through its generous support of the project on clinical narratives in breast cancer treatment, has allowed a new research paradigm to address difficult issues in cancer therapeutics. I thank these organizations for their willingness to sustain ethnographic research.

I acknowledge those in California—physicians, nurse practitioners, midwives and other clinicians, patients, and friends—who gave me insight into the politics of medical competence and who generously shared their thoughts in formal interviews and in informal conversations. The friendship of many made the California research truly engaging. In particular, I wish to thank Jayne and Rich Bush; Paul, Judy, and Katie Tichinin; Linda Rosengarten and Ron Hock; Georgia McCloskey; Mervyn and Peggy Hamlin; Marcie and Hanley Norins; Charlene and Allan Petersen; Mary Ellen Black; and Joanna Green.

Our psychiatrist colleague and friend, James T. Barter, M.D., supported the ethnographic aspects of the project with enthusiasm.

The study of medical education and the New Pathway innovations would not have been possible without the assertive encouragement of Leon Eisenberg, M.D., our department chair at the time, and the willing support of Harvard Medical School's deans, Daniel Tosteson, M.D., S. James Adelstein, M.D., and Daniel Federman, M.D., and the New Pathway faculty, in particular Gordon Moore, Susan Block, and Dan Goodenough. I am particularly grateful to the many medical students who participated in the study, committing their time to this project throughout their four years of medical education. Because so many participated and to maintain confidentiality I do not name them here, but they know that Part II of this book is dedicated to them.

The study of clinical narratives in oncology was stimulated by conversations with two Harvard oncologists, Rita Linggood, a radiotherapist, and Stuart Lind, a medical oncologist. These conversations were serendipitous, setting a path of investigation I would not have predicted earlier in my career. I thank the many patients who have participated in the current project for opening their experience and thoughtful interpretations to research; I hope our findings and educational endeavors that grow out of this work will assist others suffering from cancer and improve the therapeutic process. Many oncologists, oncology nurses, and radiation technicians at the Massachusetts General Hospital have also given much time and thoughtful consideration to the project, and their clerical staff have faciliated our efforts. Oncologists Rita Linggood, Irene Kuter, and Simon Powell (the British trio) have been particularly engaged and helpful in the Clinical Narratives in Breast Cancer study; Susann Wilkinson and Martha MacLeish Fuller have invested their energies in the project and helped me to realize the research with good humor, and Susan Grosdov has skillfully managed the budget. Cheryl Mattingly deserves special acknowledgment; our conversations about her work on emplotment and therapeutic narratives generated from her study of occupational therapists led me to interpret what I was seeing in oncology in new ways and to develop the project on Clinical Narratives in Breast Cancer. I thank her for such creative collegiality.

Many colleagues have read through drafts or chapters of this manuscript, including John Stoeckle, Rashi Fein, Eugenio Paci, Mariella Pandolfi, and David Riesman. I thank them for their time, forbearance, and encouragement. Arthur Kleinman, through his tremendous energetic investment in our community of scholars, has supported my work over the past decade; he also facilitated the funding of the project on clinical narratives in oncology, making it a reality. He engaged this manuscript and its ideas with intellectual enthusiasm and made many helpful suggestions. Leon Eisenberg cheered me on as he read the original draft, asked provocative questions, and advised greater brevity. The recommendations of Gilles Bibeau, Sharon Kaufmann, Michael Klein, and Lorna Rhodes were particularly helpful guides as I reworked the original draft and attempted to correct the flaws they identified in the original manuscript. These reviewers are generous colleagues. Martha MacLeish Fuller smoothed the preparation of the manuscript and bibliography with her excellent assistance, as did Timothy Marjoribanks with his careful reading of the text and literature searches. Anne Alach, the Department of Social Medicine librarian, kept me supplied with a steady stream of relevant articles throughout the writing of this book, and Sarah Grant assisted with literature searches on women in medicine.

Stan Holwitz supported this book and its revisions with tough sympathy; an anonymous reviewer for the press gave excellent advice; Michelle Nordon guided the production process with care and tact; and Linda Benefield carefully copyedited the manuscript.

My husband, Byron J. Good, is at the heart of this book. Together we carried out the research in California and on medical education. Our conversations about these studies and about my work on oncology inform my interpretations and arguments. Byron has read every word of this manuscript, from the moment I first began writing to its conclusion. He has been my chief critic, editor, and champion. I dedicate the completion of this book to him, with love.

Introduction

Engaging the Field

This book is about the meaning of physician competence in medical practice, medical politics, and medical education in the United States in the late twentieth century. Its central theme is an exploration of competence as a core symbol in the culture of American medicine and an examination of what competence means to individual physicians and to the profession at large.

The Emergence of a Perspective from the Research Field

In over a decade of research with physicians in primary care and specialty medicine, with medical students, and with colleagues on medical faculties, I have repeatedly encountered disquiet about the profession's eroding cultural authority and power.[1] In public forums, medical journals, and interviews, physicians express concern about the many challenges to the profession's claims to "competence" and to its authority to define and control the "quality" of health care. How should doctors be trained to attain the highest standards of medical competence, in particular without losing essential "caring" qualities expected by the public? How should the profession sustain and enhance the competence of its members in the face of extraordinary

1

transformations in biomedical knowledge and technologies? Why, when the science of medicine appears most advanced, does the political and economic organization of medical practice appear to threaten "good doctoring," collegial relationships, and adequate care of patients? Who should have the authority to decide requisite competencies in medical work and determine specialty boundaries? What should the profession's response be to rising costs of medical liability, intermittent malpractice crises, and collective responsibility for limiting harm to patients? How can the quality of medical knowledge, practice, and care be preserved when the financing and delivery of health care and the very institutions of our medical commons are in turmoil?[2] Deeply rooted in the cultural history of American medicine, this ongoing discourse about the competence of doctors has shaped, as it has been shaped by, the evolution of the profession and the health care system.

My interest in what competence means in the practice and politics of medicine emerged from field research with rural physicians which my husband and I began over a decade ago. When I first asked physicians what they found to be the most difficult aspect of rural practice, to my surprise they remarked they were most disturbed by disputes with medical colleagues over competent medical practice. "Competence" talk was constant and appeared to be the most common language used to speak about colleagues, relations among the specialties, the profession at large, and its travails with the legal system (M. Good 1985).

Throughout our study of rural medical practice, I repeatedly discovered that power struggles between general practitioners and board certified specialists in internal medicine and obstetrics were articulated in talk about the competence of colleagues and competitors. Turf battles erupted among general practitioners, family medicine physicians, midwives, and obstetricians; disagreements over who was authorized to set standards of care, practice, and review were most often voiced in highly charged debates over provider competence and, in the case of obstetrics, over ideologies of birthing. Rising malpractice insurance costs sharpened competition and debates, at times tearing the fabric of medical communities. Professional civility among members of medical staffs of rural community hospitals in the 1970s and 1980s, in particular between consultants and general practitioners, was often jeopardized. Structural changes in the organization of medical practice, including the coming of specialists to rural areas and changes in hospital governance and ownership, often generated intense disputes about what constituted competent medical care. Such debates often burst into public awareness, engaging hospital boards, medical staff, and whole communities in heated controversy.

I was captured by these first field experiences and followed these rural medical communities from 1980 to 1987 through a number of "crises of competence." As I went on to study biomedical clinician-investigators, medical education, and most recently, oncology and high-technology specialties, I found my interest in competence to have continued relevance. The talk about physician competence I found in rural medical communities appeared even more prevalent in the halls of academic medicine and medical education. Interviews with researcher-clinicians at an academic medical center revealed that cleavages between freestanding clinicians and physicians primarily engaged in bench research were framed in terms of relative clinical competence, as were battles over resources, space, and institutional prestige. These issues were by no means only of local relevance.

Robert Petersdorf, former editor of the *Annals of Internal Medicine,* wrote that "the triple threat academician is just as defunct as one platoon football" and "physicians who leave their ivory tower half a day a week or a month a year to practice clinical medicine do so poorly, unless they restrict their practice to a highly specialized area." He argued that "we are in an era of specialists" and "it is unrealistic to expect an academic to stay at the top in research for an entire career or even to remain in the same clinical field" (Petersdorf 1983:1053–1057). Clinician-researchers who aspired to what Petersdorf labeled a "defunct" role were troubled by his statements because he used "competence" to argue the comparative value of clinical investigation and clinical services, thereby threatening the role of clinician-investigator (see Stossel 1987).

Our second major study of the profession examined curricular innovations in medical education (the New Pathway) at Harvard Medical School (see B. Good 1984, chapter 3; M. Good and B. Good 1989; B. Good and M. Good 1993). The curricular reform provided fertile ground to investigate how organizational change within medical education is motivated in terms of "professional competence." Many faculty resisted the innovation. And although struggles over departmental power and influence in the educational process were often at the core of the resistance, faculty debates were framed in terms of how best to create competent physicians. Students were attuned to faculty opposition, and "competence" talk came readily to the fore.

In spontaneous discussions in tutorials and classes and in private interviews, students anxiously questioned whether the new curriculum (problem-based and student-oriented learning) would really prepare them to become competent physicians, to have the requisite knowledge and skills appropriate to begin clinical training. Critical comments of faculty opposed to the new curriculum raised for students the ominous possibility of "medical incompetence." Nevertheless, as the study progressed over five years, I became most interested in the social creation of medical "competence" through clinical training, in how students learn to become competent physicians, through presenting patients and performing for the training team, and finally through crafting purposive clinical narratives with consequences for patient care.

In my current research on oncology, my interest in competence has shifted from a focus on professional interactions to exploring how oncologists shape competent clinical narratives for and with patients. In this setting, competence is defined as joining the two worlds of oncology, the science and the therapeutics. Clinical work and patient care must respond to constantly evolving treatment technologies and scientific uncertainties. In the perspective of these oncologists, a competent clinical narrative arises from routine technologies used in new ways and from uncertainties about the efficacy of treatments and of the biomedical sciences that underpin the clinical craft.

Throughout my research, physicians and medical students have reflected on what competence means to them. Students have spoken about experiences in the study of biosciences and clinical training that enhanced their sense of becoming competent physicians and about situations that were detrimental to their professional development. Physicians related how their vision of professional competence informs their practice and professional ethics and influences their relationships with patients and colleagues. Clinicians have told me how they contend with their own errors or those of their colleagues, with medical mishaps, bad judgment, and unavoidable "acts of God" that lead to the death or harm of patients. These conversations reveal frustrations physicians experience not only with medical-legal institutions and with medical malpractice, but with the limitations of peer review and educational processes. They indicate why an assault on one's competence, provoked by the unexpected death of a patient, a malpractice suit, or a colleague's critical review, can be shattering. In these conversations professional concerns about becoming and being competent clinicians are wed to life histories and personal values. These interviews also reflect our society's debates over what it means to be a good doctor in an era when the profession is under intense public scrutiny and resources are limited.[3]

Engaging the Disciplinary Traditions

Although my initial field studies generated the questions and ideas about medical competence I subsequently developed in a series of essays and turn to in this book, when I first began the research with rural physicians I found myself comparing my interpretations of what I was observing with the classic arguments from medical sociology about knowledge and professional power (Parsons 1978; Freidson 1970a, 1970b, 1975, 1986, 1989). Although theoretical discourses on the medical profession have greatly expanded since the classic work of Talcott Parsons and Eliot Freidson, the relations of power and knowledge they addressed continue to command our attention. Parsons wrote his first essays on the profession in the 1950s, when social regard for physicians was remarkably high. Exploring the source of the special fiduciary relationship of physicians and patients, he defined what empirically constituted professional competence. Patients should be able to presume that physicians possessed high intelligence and moral character, technical knowledge and skills acquired through formal education in the basic sciences and clinical training, and a responsibility and willingness to act as genuine trustees for their health interests (Parsons 1978). These characteristics still hold sway today in medical education and practice as broad measures of the empirical competence of physicians.

In the 1970s, Freidson brought a far more critical perspective to the study of medicine and examined the profession's dominance over the content and context of medical work. He questioned society's presumption of medical competence and drew our attention to the profession's "conspiracy of silence" regarding the incompetence of colleagues and its failure to engage in aggressive peer review, perhaps foretelling the decline of patient trust characteristic of recent decades.

Neither of these classical interpretations, however, explained what I was seeing in the field in 1982 and in 1994. The "conspiracy of silence" had clearly been pierced in the medical communities I studied, although in certain contexts silence and ambiguity could be found and formal peer review was often flawed. And while professional talk about competence referred to physicians' knowledge, technical skills, judgment, and moral character, it conveyed many other meanings as well. The inherent uncertainties and risks of bioscience and clinical practice identified by Renee Fox (1988) in over a generation of studies on medical education, practice, and experimental research, challenged the assumption that professional competence was grounded on a bedrock of empirical knowledge and technical skill.

The shifts in disciplinary discourses and interpretative paradigms have been considerable in the decade since I first began to write about physician competence. Although current assessments of the state of the profession continue to draw on classic sociological concepts in debates about professional dominance, proletarianization, or corporate control over quality of care (Light and Levine 1988; McKinlay 1988; Mechanic 1994; Navarro 1988; Stoeckle 1988), classical interpretations about medicine's power and knowledge have been superseded by numerous nuanced ethnographies from sociologists and anthropologists working in diverse theoretical traditions. These studies of medical knowledge, training, and practice, now part of the current conversation on the culture and political economy of contemporary American medicine, highlight the limits of both classical and current writings that characterize the medical profession in largely monolithic terms— as "biomedicine" or "Western medicine" (see Bosk 1979; B. Good 1994; Light 1980; Hahn and Gaines 1985; Kleinman 1988a, Lindenbaum and Lock 1993; Lock and Gordon 1988; Martin 1987; Mizrahi 1986; Rhodes 1991, among others). They have also transformed our theoretical discourses about medicine—from feminist theorizing on the gendered structure of medical knowledge and power, to analyses of the medical gaze, surveillance, and monitoring which have been profoundly influenced by the work of Foucault (Arney 1982; Davis-Floyd 1992; Haraway 1993; Martin 1987 and 1993; Rabinow 1993; Treichler 1992). Ultimately, these studies caution against presenting an overly unified picture of the profession or professional discourse as we explore the culture of competence in American medicine today.

Facets and Puzzles

Rather than pursue a single ethnographic story or linear argument, this book approaches the study of physician competence as a puzzle to be assembled from several ethnographic and analytic perspectives. Each ethnographic study and analysis of parallel national trends is designed to illuminate a facet of the culture of competence in American medicine. Each is motivated by the broad question of how competence becomes the core symbol in American medicine for individual physicians and for professional collectivities.[4] And each focuses not only on the culture of competence but on professional power and institutional contexts within which the meanings of medical competence are produced and negotiated.

More specific questions generated from experiences in the field focus these explorations: Why does talk about competent and incompetent physicians generate such passion within medicine and in our broader culture? What do professional discussions about competence imply about hierarchical relationships among communities of physicians, about collective responsibility for standards of practice and care, about liability and the recent crises in malpractice? Why do we find widespread professional concern about medical competence in certain contexts but observe professional silences about medical errors in others? How do flurries of internal professional critique relate to transformations in the organization of our health care system and in our institutions of medical education and patient care? What is revealed about gender and power structures in the local worlds of medical practice and medical education when viewed through the lens of physician competence? How do extraordinary advances in the biosciences and medical technology bear upon how competence is constituted by different medical specialties?

The first chapter, "Medical Malpractice and the Voices of Medicine," presents a picture of the ferment over medical liability and malpractice that colored the period throughout the ethnographic studies. The ways individual physicians and medical collectivities responded to the malpractice crises illustrate a diversity of professional voices and repertoires of discourse on competence. I conclude this introduction with an analytic frame for disaggregating these multiple voices and for aiding our thinking about the social contexts and political purposes reflected in these distinct discourses on medical competence.

Three ethnographic parts follow, each addressing a facet of the puzzle. "The Transformations of the Culture of Competence in Rural Medicine: Contests of Specialty and Gender" (chapters 2–5) is based on the study of primary care physicians and obstetricians in rural practice and explores how, in everyday clinical life, competence articulates changing relations of specialty power within medical communities and the gendering of medical knowledge and practice. I recount the historical roots and evolution of a local crisis of competence and conclude with an analysis of the national crisis in obstetrics and medical malpractice to contextualize the local experience in larger social processes.

"The Quest for Competence through Medical Education" (chapters 6 and 7) explores how students learn medicine in an institutional context of educational innovation, eventually developing competence in crafting clinical narratives and finding a "moral" professional voice. "Culture, Competence, and Clinical Science" (chapter 8) focuses on the practice of oncology and examines how specialty concepts about competence are institutionalized in the clinical narratives and narrative strategies created for patients which are intended to join the two worlds of uncertain science and therapeutics with patient care. The Epilogue, "The Relevance of Competence to Policy" (chapter 9) addresses the link between competence and political economy and suggests ways of conceptualizing competence that bear upon research and policy in medical education, specialist-generalist relationships, and clinical narratives in high-technology specialties, such as oncology. And because the cultural authority of American medicine has a global reach, I conclude with an international perspective on the meaning of competence.

It is my hope that this book will not only contribute to our understanding of the culture of American medicine as it is currently practiced and taught but will also provide insights from ethnographic research useful to those engaged in formulating new policies in medical education and training, professional ethics, and health care reforms as they shape the culture and political economy of the profession into the twenty-first century.

CHAPTER ONE

Medical Malpractice and the Voices of Medicine

An individual physician's biomedical knowledge and clinical skills provide the primary referent for the *symbol* "medical competence." However, a careful look at the world of medicine quickly reveals that the language of "competence" bears within it the practical activities of which it is a part, and the "contexts in which it has lived its intense social life" (Mikhail Bakhtin, in Todorov 1984:56–57).[1] Competence is not only an "empirical reality," an attribute of physicians, but a core symbol that mediates a variety of experiences and carries diverse meanings. Doctors speak about how feelings of professional competence fluctuate throughout their professional lives, how their sense of competence is often dependent on context and influenced by the medical community within which they practice, actions of the profession at large, and crises and events that often entail public scrutiny. But physicians also identify the core of their professional identity with an "essential" competence in their knowledge and practice of medicine. Professional competence is thus subject to advances in the biosciences and technologies, as well as to competing philosophies concerning standards of practice and care, and ultimately to power relationships within the profession.

Cultural and social studies of science and technology have addressed how symbolic products of science should be used to explore the production and reproduction of a particular science, its producers, and its claims to knowledge (Traweek 1993:10). Sharon Traweek, in a review of diverse theoretical and methodological strategies in this field,

9

identifies the cultural studies of interpretive anthropologists as attending, in particular, "to patterned interactions, such as oral and written discourses, or any other 'social text'"—from an article, to a conference, a policy or set of terms, and even a poem. Traweek argues that "discursive, strategic, evocative practices are key terms" to explore "how relations of power are enacted/performed/reproduced locally and globally through discursive practices/representations/evocations" (1993:11).

Noted British sociologists of science have also encouraged exploring the diversity of repertoires of discourse in science, to assemble from the "radically different, yet quite plausible" stories (Mulkay 1981: 170) of "how that science really is" (Mulkay et al. 1983:196), how "scientists' discourse is organized to convey varying conceptions of scientific action and belief on different occasions and in different contexts" (Mulkay and Gilbert 1982b:588–589). Natural scientists, argue Michael Mulkay and G. N. Gilbert, primarily draw on "empiricist" and "contingent" repertoires. They generally describe their own work in public and in the research literature in empiricist terms in which science is treated as the logical discovery of "the facts" of the natural world. In contrast, when called on to account for errors in scientific disputes, they often blame those errors on contingent factors, and science is presented as much less uniform, subject to personal and social factors, to intuition and practical skills (Mulkay and Gilbert 1982b).

When we examine the discursive interactions of contemporary American medicine, such as the profession's responses to the medical liability crises, problems similar to those encountered in social and cultural studies of science appear evident. Contradictory representations of medical practice emerge, depending on whose words in what contexts are examined. Disaggregating the repertoires of discourse on physician competence produced by the medical profession allows us to clarify the social and political roots of these apparent contradictions.[2]

The multiple voices of the profession present in the malpractice debates suggest three primary repertoires in which physicians speak and write about competence: (1) an intra-professional repertoire primarily internal to and intended only for members of the profession; (2) an extra-professional repertoire consciously designed to represent professional interests and to mediate between medicine and the public; and (3) a reflective repertoire, providing individual physicians with acceptable cultural genres through which to explore experiences of competence and incompetence. Each repertoire is produced by particular social contexts, informed by specific logics, audiences, and intended actions. Employing these three analytic categories encourages a disaggregation of popular presentations of medicine's monolithic voice, enabling us to include conflicting opinions and diverse modes of speaking and writing about competence within a single analytic frame.[3]

Analyzing the social uses of these repertoires also provokes questions about why one genre is culturally permissible in particular professional contexts but negatively sanctioned in others. Negative sanctions turn our focus not only to the social and hierarchical contexts within which different repertoires are produced but also to how critiques of physician competence are given a normative shape, appearing as power-laden and rule-governed. When discussions of incompetence appear strikingly beyond traditional norms but are accommodated in new ways, broader transformations in the organization of the profession or in the content of professional knowledge appear implicated.

The Medical Liability Debate and Medicine's Multiple Voices

The medical liability crises of the 1970s and 1980s colored medical politics and finances in a fashion previously unencountered in the United States. Although malpractice costs and claims had risen rather precipitously in the 1970s, the increases in the 1980s were of such magnitude as to shock the profession and the public into a serious review of causes and consequences. In simple numerical terms, the cost of medical liability insurance had risen from approximately $2.5 billion in 1983 to a peak of $7 billion in 1988, and although the costs in real dollar amounts declined in the 1990s, medical liability insurance accounted for 1 percent of total costs of health care in 1993 (Roberts 1993:133).

Perhaps most striking was the increase in the rate of malpractice claims against physicians. The demise of the "golden era of trust" between patients and physicians of midcentury is documented through the extraordinary rise in malpractice claims. Claims rose from one per hundred doctors in 1960 to a peak of seventeen per hundred doctors in 1988, dropping to thirteen per hundred physicians by the end of the decade.[4] Rises in the claim rates against obstetricians over the three decades were even more astonishing.[5] The dramatic increases in claim rates and medical liability costs represent a larger story about transformations in the practice of medicine and in the relationship between the profession and the public. How individual physicians and professional groups responded to the challenges to professional competence embedded in these debates presents one facet of this larger story.

Collective and Individual Responses to Malpractice

The malpractice suit strikes at the whole core of your competence, at the core of your effectiveness, of your honesty. It's a very personal thing to physicians.

(Practicing physician, in Harvard Medical Practice Study 1990:9–57)

We must remember that the liability crisis is not confined to being a problem of bad medicine. . . . [T]he administration of health care to persons who are not well will always carry inherent risks, but . . . most health care providers are competently delivering quality health care to the vast majority of patients. . . .

Over the past decade, the profession has vigorously addressed these system issues under several rubrics. . . . All aim at the common goal of preventing patient injury. All call upon us to examine what we do or fail to do, and how we do it. . . .

These efforts clearly represent a new era in the medical community's ability to respond aggressively to patient safety concerns. It should be noted that the frequency of medical liability claims filings appears to have stabilized and, in some states even decreased since approximately 1986.

(J. S. Todd, Executive Vice President, American Medical Association, in Campion 1990:xiv, xv, xvii)

Physicians traditionally have resisted standards of practice that prescribe specific details of their day-to-day conduct of medical care.

(J. H. Eichorn, in Eichorn et al. 1990:76)

Medical care is a hazardous enterprise, the injuries inflicted on patients are real and painful.

(Paul C. Weiler, in Weiler 1991:16)

Among the many consequences of the medical liability crises has been a striking if discreet reexamination *by representatives within the medical community* of how physicians practice medicine and the association of particular practices with rates of medical accidents, malpractice claims, and costs of liability insurance. The technological and institutional contexts of medical care have also come under new forms of professional evaluation. The first three comments by physicians noted above represent ways the profession has sought to make sense of the sea change in medical practice and liability. The first comment is an example of a reflective and private discourse—the response of an individual physician interviewed in a research context. The second and third comments are taken from publications by physicians, designed primarily for an audience of physicians; however, the authors recognize that this is public discourse that may be reviewed by the legal profession or by patients. The fourth quotation, by the noted legal scholar Paul Weiler, expresses the public concern about medicine as a hazardous enterprise, representing one aspect of the conversation about medical practice and malpractice that is ongoing among physicians, lawyers, and patients. The logic of each of the arguments suggested in these comments and the audiences for whom they are intended are discussed below.

When extraordinary rises in malpractice costs first began to shock physicians in the early 1980s, the popular media stepped in to cover the protests of physicians and the concerns of patients. Doctors threatened to restrict their practices, many obstetricians and family physicians who delivered babies ceased doing so, and state medical societies appealed for legislative reforms. Physicians blamed the crisis on failures in the fault-based system of tort law; in more passionate moments they accused lawyers and insurance companies of greed, and argued that patients had unrealistic expectations of medicine's power to cure and care. These complaints were directed to the public and to legislatures as well as to colleagues.

When physicians initially turned to examine themselves, they occasionally faulted their relationships with patients, their failure to create trust and properly explain to patients the limits and risks of medical care. They declared that changes in the social environment of medical practice were the root causes of the malpractice crisis, not the incompetence of professionals. And they pointed to examples—the general increase in public skepticism about medicine (and all the professions) and a decline in the public trust, perhaps due to the commercialization of medicine (Relman 1990).[6] In these early protests to the public, physicians did not speak about professional competence, clinical standards, medical accidents, and medical negligence. Rather they spoke about medical uncertainty, unavoidable hazards and risks of high-technology medicine, and about redesigning physician-patient relationships. This was a language about "the soft side of medicine," about problems with the art of medicine as practiced in the late twentieth century.

In response to these early ad hoc protests, the American Medical Association, specialty societies, the Institute of Medicine, and other professional and academic groups took a highly aggressive approach to dealing with what they termed the medical liability crisis. This shift in professional terminology—from malpractice to liability crisis—appears to represent a reformulation of the problem from bad practice to runaway costs and problems with trust. Professional organizations picked up the popular complaints of individual physicians and lobbied for legislative interventions and legal reform. Yet they also introduced a series of activities intended to preserve the power and autonomy of the profession to regulate itself. Many of these activities came to be viewed by some doctors as challenges to the practice autonomy of individual physicians.

Programs in "risk management" and "quality assurance," designed to reduce the cost of liability insurance by reducing variability in the quality of medical practice, opened the way to develop written practice standards and clinical guidelines.[7] Such activities addressed the "hard side of medicine" or how one should use scientific and biomedical knowledge and techniques in everyday work. This consideration, new to many specialties, has drawn renewed attention to how competently physicians practice, the quality of the technical products they use, and the standards of care in the institutional settings within which they work. Clearly, the profession has launched a new era of self-regulation and review. Some efforts have been labeled as such—for example the "Agenda for Change" introduced in 1987 by the Joint Commission on Accreditation of Healthcare Organizations (Todd 1990:xvii).[8]

Although the profession has turned to examine itself and its standards of practice in new ways, many physicians have been reluctant to identify professional incompetence as a significant cause of malpractice cases and rising liability costs, even when they are willing to acknowledge the need to improve practice standards. There are complex reasons why physicians appear to resist an interpretation that links incompetence to negligence and malpractice—and why the legal system finds it not at all difficult to make this link.

A LEGAL VOICE

Weiler, a professor of law at Harvard, reminds us in his important critique of our American fault-based tort system, *Medical Malpractice on Trial* (1991), that medical accidents are due to the momentary inattention and carelessness of physicians and other health care providers, and that these "accidents" are bound to occur in the context of high-technology medical practice. He remarks on the limitations of medical licensing, its focus on the "especially poor doctor," and its inability effectively to "define and enforce appropriate standards of care for the average doctor" (1991:110). Weiler argues:

If the medical accident problem were largely attributable to a few bad apples in the profession, this single minded emphasis would make some sense. But the sources of iatrogenic injuries are widespread. These injuries are the outgrowth of techniques and mishaps of generally conscientious doctors who must function in a highly risky and unforgiving physical environment. Therefore, more sophisticated policy instruments are required to reduce the chance of errors and to minimize the harm when they occur. Traditional medical licensing is simply not designed for this ambitious role. (1991:222)

Weiler frequently refers to "careless" doctors throughout his text,[9] and to "inattention" that leads to accidents and medical negligence; however, he generally does so without a weighty judgment of moral "wrongdoing." Yet he acknowledges that for physicians, a malpractice suit may be experienced as "the more dramatic morality play of tort litigation" (1991:149), that it entails a "quasi-moral judgment" about "poor performance" (1991:148). Weiler proposes consideration of a no-fault alternative for compensating patients; such a system, he argues, not only would be able to compensate a greater number of patients who suffer iatrogenic injuries but would disengage compensation for medical accidents from the emotional aspects of tort suits (1991: see chapters 5, 6).

The linkage of "accidents" to "carelessness," "negligence," and "incompetence" (however momentary) is fundamental to our tort system of redress for iatrogenic injuries to patients. For physicians, however, such a linkage appears far more problematic. Comments by physicians interviewed as part of the Harvard Medical Practice Study indicate some reasons for their resistance to this linkage.[10]

THE REFLECTIVE VOICE
OF INDIVIDUAL DOCTORS

*I think it's bad judgment, not negligence; people make
wrong decisions after consideration. You know—after
careful consideration of the facts you can make what turns
out to be a bad decision; that's clearly not negligence.*

(Harvard Medical Practice Study 1990:9–49)

Forty-seven physicians—surgeons, internists, and obstetricians—were interviewed at length for the Harvard Medical Practice Study. All commented on a series of case scenarios specific to their specialty that included examples of substandard care and harm to or death of patients. Those who had had a malpractice claim brought against them also were invited to speak about their experiences with the tort system.

A disturbing confusion in physicians' comments on competence and malpractice emerged both in discussions about case scenarios and in accounts of their own medical malpractice experiences. Although most physicians readily identified errors and substandard care in the case scenarios they reviewed, they discriminated between "medical mistakes" and physician incompetence and negligence (Harvard Medical Practice Study 1990: chap. 9). Medical judgments that created iatrogenic injuries and adverse outcomes were not necessarily attributed to physician incompetence, carelessness, or negligence, nor regarded as warranting compensation.

The authors of the project interpreted the reluctance of both internists and surgeons to associate medical mismanagement and errors to negligence and incompetence as a reluctance to equate medical mistakes with an *intent* to practice poor medicine, to err morally. In summarizing the interviews, they wrote,

The internists expressed much stronger disagreements on the finding of negligence than on the finding of a deviation from the standard of care or a definite error. The causation question, however, provoked the most controversy amongst internists. A finding of causation was not as clear-cut for these physicians as it was for the surgeons. Again, the physicians were confused about negligence and reluctant to compensate for iatrogenic injury. (1990: chap. 9, p. 51)

Although surgeons followed a different logic in identifying errors and mistakes, they too were regarded by the research team as having problems in judging negligence. Surgeons do not equate failure to meet the standard of care with negligence. Rather they seem to believe negligence requires culpability beyond the standard of care threshold. . . . Most physicians believe they are competent. Even so, they realize they can make mistakes. The label of negligence, however, appears to make physicians feel as if they were incompetent. (1990: chap. 9, p. 45)

The obstetricians/gynecologists were more explicit about errors, malpractice, and physicians' financial accountability, perhaps indicating greater familiarity with tort law. Obstetricians also "evidence a greater consistency between their judgments regarding the standard of care, error and negligence" in their case reviews (1990: chap. 9, p. 55).

Physicians who had had malpractice claims brought against them ranged from seeing these suits as "distractions" or "an expected consequence of practicing medicine in the litigious climate" to describing a profound sense of hurt and "assault" (1990: chap. 9, p. 57). The physician quoted above who remarked that a suit "strikes at the whole core of your competence, at the core of your effectiveness, of your honesty" (1990: chap. 9, p. 57) spoke to the moral culpability implied by the suit. Others recalled the frustrations of malpractice trials: "The lawyer's whole aim was to try to show me as an incompetent fool . . . it's extremely frustrating to hear these statements made and not be able to refute them" and the lawyer's attitude was " 'It's all business . . . nothing personal, it's all business.' Well it *is* personal, and to physicians it is *not* business" (1990: chap. 9, p. 58). The moral interpretations physicians gave to these suits, if taken at face value, suggest the different meanings doctors and lawyers attribute to incompetence and negligence and highlight the clash between these two professional cultures.

Physicians regard "findings of single episodes of negligence as tantamount to judgments of incompetence" and an attack on their professional morality (1990: chap. 9, p. 66).[11] In law, negligence identifies the quality of the physician's action *at the time of treatment,* an action that may be regarded as "incompetent."[12] Weiler's discussion of the American tort system emphasizes this perspective as he refers to iatrogenic injuries as "medical accidents." In medicine, as illustrated by the physicians' comments on the case scenarios and on being sued, a legal finding of negligence may be perceived as a judgment about one's *essential* competence rather than about specific and momentary actions. References to carelessness also suggest intent through omission, and therefore a moral failure to uphold one's responsibility as a physician, rather than an unintended and momentary mistake. The apparent reluctance of some physicians to label substandard care as negligence becomes far more understandable in light of these different meanings that "negligence" conveys in law and in medicine.

Words carry meanings from the places where they have been used, and their social history is never absent from a particular usage (Mikhail Bakhtin, in Todorov 1984). The association of medical negligence with essential incompetence and with behavior regarded as professionally immoral conveys a threat that is ingrained during medical training and derived from the culture of medicine rather than from the legal system. When physicians reflect on competence in private, their conflating of the momentary with the essential and their fear of confounding medical mistakes with essential incompetence and moral culpability become apparent. This confusion motivates resistance to equating medical mistakes with legal and compensatable negligence.

The responses of organized medicine regarding negligence and medical liability follow quite a different logic than those of individual physicians. Official policies, journal essays, and conferences on "risk management," "quality assurance," and "clinical practice standards" directly address the link between medical accidents and negligence. Professional collectivities of physicians, from specialty societies to academic clinicians, appear far less hesitant to identify these linkages, and they evidence remarkably little reluctance to address incompetence as one source of the medical liability crisis. The political and financial interests of the profession to control standards of practice and to reduce the cost of malpractice motivate the logic of collective discourses on competence that have evolved into a new era of professional review.

A New Era: The Discourse on Collective Responsibility

James S. Todd, M.D., the executive vice president of the American Medical Association, in *Grand Rounds on Medical Malpractice* (Campion 1990), noted that the medical profession's efforts of the past decade to address the malpractice crisis "represent a new era in the medical community's ability to respond aggressively to patient safety concerns" (Campion 1990:xvii). James F. Holzer, a lawyer and until recently vice president of loss prevention, Risk Management Foundation of the Harvard Medical Institutions, also remarked on the "relatively new phenomenon" of efforts to devise "risk-control standards" applicable to clinical practice (Campion 1990:92). Both Todd and Holzer, representative spokesmen for organized medicine and for medicine's legal power, were referring to the flurry of collective actions taken in response to the medical liability crisis by the profession's specialty societies, the American Medical Association, physician-owned insurance carriers, and even medical staff of hospitals and other health care institutions.

The actions that initiated this "new era" included efforts to reduce the risk of harm to patients, mitigate the possibilities for physician negligence, and reduce the risk of malpractice suits and the cost of liability. Nascent efforts to develop and publish clinical guidelines and practice standards, aimed at reducing liability costs through reducing patient harm and physician risk of malpractice, are among the most striking innovations of the profession's effort to reshape the face of medical liability.[13] And although the states and the federal government initiated legislation to enhance institutional peer review and quality assurance, medicine's professional organizations aggressively sought to recover the lead in these domains. What was new about these activities?

When leaders of the medical profession write commentaries for rank-and-file physicians on the medical liability crisis and promote efforts of organized medicine to counter the crisis, they often begin with a *disclaimer,* an *acknowledgment,* and an *argument* (see Relman 1989; Campion 1990:xiii–xix). *Grand Rounds on Medical Malpractice* (Campion 1990), a casebook designed to offer "high quality instruction for physicians on the complex issues of medical malpractice," illustrates this logic.[14] In the introduction, Todd begins with a disclaimer that neither incompetence nor negligence is implicated in the dramatic rise in medical liability costs. He acknowledges that medical care has inherent risks for patients, and that physicians, even the best and most competent, make mistakes. He argues that the tort system is "broken," requiring a new physician-patient alliance to bring about reform. He writes:

Physicians are often sued not because they are negligent, but because they practice an imperfect science. . . . It is by now well documented that all doctors, even the best doctors, can and do make mistakes. (Campion 1990:xv)

The tort system needs to be fixed to meet the needs of the real parties at interest, patients and health care providers. . . . [T]he fact remains that when our patients are convinced that physicians care about their safety, and that reform proposals are fair, the possibility exists for more effective physician-patient alliances. (xviii–xix)

These comments, like others generated by risk management and peer review projects, are oriented to an audience of rank-and-file physicians presumed to be highly sensitive to equating incompetence with the medical liability crisis. The rank and file are also thought to be resistant to incursions—even by their own professional organizations—on individual autonomy in clinical work. Promoting new efforts at professional self-regulation requires a balancing act, one able to disarm doctors' traditional resistance to regulation, defuse protests against encroachment on clinical autonomy, and distance the moral and judgmental dimensions of critiques of customary practices. Organized medicine reached into its cultural history to argue that if the profession does not take the lead, its power and authority for self-regulation will be eroded by actions of the state, the legal community, and insurers (Eichorn et al. 1990; Weiler 1991). Although professional activities in risk management may be creating a new phenomenon of professional regulation and review, they also continue the profession's historical traditions of aggressively preserving professional autonomy.

The new phenomena of risk management and programs in developing additional clinical guidelines and standards ("standard mania") pose an intriguing challenge to many in the medical profession. These programs not only address the very *essence* of professional competence, they also shift the primary locus of authority to define what constitutes competent practice beyond the boundaries of local medical communities to national specialty and professional groups. They also focus on collective responsibility and the limits in the practice and knowledge of the professional collectivity.[15] Specialty groups have readily advocated more rigorous guidelines for practice standards, although recommendations are sugar-coated by appeals to the loftier ideals of patient safety and high medical competence as well as to the profession's desired goal to reduce malpractice claims and costs.

Discourses on Risk and Standards

The projects that led to the promulgation of national specialty standards of care in the 1980s earned the label "standard mania" (Holzer 1990:83–84). An example from anesthesiology serves to illustrate how this particular version of a professional discourse on competence becomes inscribed in clinical practice standards.

In August, 1986, the Department of Anesthesia at Harvard Medical

School published "specific, detailed, mandatory standards for minimal patient monitoring during anesthesia" in the *Journal of the American Medical Association* (see Campion 1990:76–81, where these standards were reprinted). These were "the first written patient-monitoring standards developed primarily to control professional liability claims" (Holzer 1990:82) and were based on a review of cases of major morbidity or death, most of which were judged as preventable with more meticulous patient monitoring. The authors expected resistance to their recommendation for mandatory national standards—a model "valid for all of American medicine" (Eichern et al., 1990:81). They crafted their recommendations to address the tradition of local practice autonomy, to disarm accusations and the fear of "big brotherism." They wrote:

Physicians traditionally have resisted standards of practice that prescribe specific details of their day-to-day conduct of medical care. . . . Standards such as these have not previously existed at Harvard. Reported herein is the process used to balance physician autonomy in daily practice with the large general goal of improving patient care, which, in turn, should mitigate the malpractice crisis. (Eichorn et al. 1990:76)

Appealing to the tradition of residency training that historically has promulgated standards of care, the authors argued that "standards in medical care take many forms . . . [as do] criteria for clinical teaching or clinical skills." Resistance in terms of limited technology was addressed: "opinions and practices in medicine vary among institutions and regions," and basic and minimal standards can be developed that focus on "behavior and habits" rather than on "expensive technology" (Eichorn et al., 1990:80). The authors concluded that mandatory minimal standards were accepted with "minimal resistance" because they avoided "major or disruptive mandated changes in practice." By 1989, the decline in anesthesia accidents, injuries, claims, and liability premiums appeared to confirm the group's work, as premium rates dropped to one-half the 1985 costs and one-third the 1988 costs (Holzer 1990:84).

The Harvard anesthesiology example is but one of the many recent efforts to develop clinically based standards designed for risk management. The general response of organized medicine has been that it is far preferable for professional groups to devise clinical standards and guidelines than to resist, only to be subjected to guidelines that are neither voluntary nor physician-generated but dictated by insurance carriers or by state regulatory boards.[16] This desire to maintain control over the definition of clinical standards has led a number of specialty societies to develop more specific practice guidelines, despite the dismay of some individual clinicians. A recent tabulation counted seven hundred practice guideline projects with twenty-six physician groups engaged in these efforts, which have also earned congressional support (Garnick, Hendricks, and Brennan 1991:2857). Practice guideline projects extend the role of the medical societies in defining domains of competence in everyday clinical work. As individual clinicians fret about the loss of professional practice autonomy in response to these emerging clinical standards, the diversity of voices and of discourses on competence is highlighted. It is not surprising therefore that practice guidelines and specialty standards have been subject to criticism. The assessment of their effectiveness in reducing medical accidents and malpractice suits is being closely monitored by medicine's rank and file (ibid. 1991).

This "new era" has fostered some extraordinary studies of malpractice, such as the Harvard Medical Practice Study (1990; Weiler et al. 1993), and serious evaluations of peer review and quality assurance in our society's institutions of health care. It has also generated a thoughtful examination of the ethical and medicolegal arrangements that shape our culture's institutions of medicine and health care (Weiler 1991; Brennan 1991).

Three Repertoires on Competence

The medical liability crises of the 1980s profoundly influenced how physicians spoke and wrote about medical competence. These discursive practices, as well as observations from my field research, informed the analytic frame of the three repertoires of discourse on competence (see M. Good 1985). This analytic perspective has equal relevance for understanding relations of power in the everyday worlds of clinical practice and medical education and for interpreting how the profession produces and reproduces the meanings of physician competence through its diverse voices.

THE INTRA-PROFESSIONAL VOICE

Physicians frequently talk among themselves about colleagues whose inadequacies are a source of concern. These conversations refer to deficiencies in knowledge, expertise, and clinical skills, and at times to the moral failings of doctors for whom one may have legal responsibility or joint collective liability. Although many physicians are reluctant to "cast this stone," medical mishaps and even incompetence and negligence may be identified. In this internalist repertoire, physicians "break the conspiracy of silence" about the limitations of a colleague's competence because the audience is presumed to be members of the professional community.

The language that is used to refer to the medical competence of individuals or groups of physicians may also carry another message. Competence discourse can be a powerful vehicle through which specialty cleavages and conflicts within medical communities are articulated and increased competition reflecting changes in the political economy of medical practice is expressed. Generated by rank-and-file practitioners, medical school faculty and researchers, spokespersons for the profession, and specialty societies and associations, this intra-professional repertoire may be directed to local or national audiences. For example, medical gossip, rumors among medical staff, and contests over hierarchy and power within communities of physicians are not only informal but typically local, whereas quality assurance and peer review are more formal local examples. Ideological conflicts between specialty groups over what constitutes the "best standards of competence and care"—such as debates between the specialties of obstetrics and family medicine over birthing practices—are expressed in both local and national arenas. Conflicts between specialties are carried out formally through journal articles and programs of research and education. Locally, such contests emerge informally in the context of medical practice, as through competition over the control of obstetrical practice.

Crossing the boundaries between the formal and the informal— that is, saying in a formal context what is usually said only in private— may lead to collegial sanctions. Sanctions lend the appearance of a profession maintaining a conspiracy of silence, providing evidence of professional dominance and medicine acting in its own interests. The rules for how to engage in competence talk are rigorously taught and enforced. For example, when medical students are instructed not to record disagreements with attendings or residents over patient care in a medical chart but to raise them in conversation, they are shown how and when they may raise questions that bear upon the competence of peers and attendings. They also learn about the medicolegal consequences of such actions if their formal criticisms spill into the public or legal domain.

THE PUBLIC AND
EXTRA-PROFESSIONAL VOICE

Physicians write and speak about medical competence for public as well as professional consumption. This repertoire is intended to affect public actions, such as legislative, medical liability, or financing reforms. Characteristically formal, such discourses are generated by organized medicine, specialty societies, institutions of medical education and research, quasi-governmental organizations such as the Institute of Medicine, and foundations broadly concerned with medical education and medical practice (such as the Robert Wood Johnson Foundation). Locally, the public repertoire may be mobilized to seek community support for hospital staffing policies or reforms in financing the cost of malpractice insurance. When medical communities are stressed by increased competition or changes in the financing and organization of health care, extra-professional discourses may appear less "rational" as physicians attempt to engage supporters and influence local outcomes, often by bringing into public view critiques of medical competence normally regarded as appropriate only for the professional community.

Extra-professional discourses on competence, such as discussions of risk management and clinical guidelines, are also employed by specialty groups or political collectivities, such as the AMA, with the intent of preserving the profession's dominance over the content of medical work. Nevertheless, as exemplified by responses to the malpractice crises, such collective or corporate discourses may be regarded by individual physicians as detrimental to their practice autonomy. The interest of collectivities of physicians, the health care institutions in which they practice, and the insurance carriers, many of which are physician owned, as represented in these public discourses, may therefore be in opposition to interests of individual clinicians and the profession's rank and file.[17]

THE REFLECTIVE VOICE

When physicians speak and write about anguish over medical mistakes and guilt and anger associated with challenges to their competence, or when they recall experiences of power when deft therapeutic acts made a real difference for patients, they convey why competence carries such symbolic power in medicine. Physicians use both private and public "voices" to reflect on this aspect of their professional being, and a genre of writing about competence appears in essays in professional journals and in popular doctor-authored books.

Many physicians readily talk about what medical competence means to them in terms of their own life histories and professional experiences. During my research interviews, doctors and medical students often worked through what constitutes the good physician, drawing on our society's current cultural debates on humanism and technology and on competence and gender. And they struggled with how to interpret "the bad outcomes" attributed to medical mistakes and accidents, and "the untoward outcomes" attributed to "acts of God" and unalterable disease processes. Many also discussed their discomfort or rage when they encounter the incompetence of colleagues and their pain when confronting the limits of their own competence (although none admitted to being essentially incompetent doctors). These interviews begin to uncover how physicians internalize professional self-regulation and monitoring and the sources for flaws that exist in this highly individualistic mode of self-review.

The public reflective voice of physicians, as presented in published work, is more cautious and less explicit than private conversations. For example, discussions of "the impaired physician"—considered incompetent in an essential way—take on a therapeutic if moralistic tone and convey an image of a depersonalized abstract type. "The bad apples," a less formal image, is popularly used to refer to "the few" incompetent doctors who bring unsavory publicity to the profession. Nevertheless this reflective but public genre includes personal accounts in which physicians either lay bare their own errors or those of professional colleagues.

Two recent examples illustrate this public repertoire of reflective discourse and the dangers and risks for those who engage in it. In a classic essay published in the *New England Journal of Medicine* in 1984, "Facing Our Mistakes," a rural physician recounted the circumstances surrounding his own medical errors and lamented the cultural ethos of the profession that prohibits physicians from admitting mistakes, making them fearful of bringing "medical mistakes out of the closet" (Hilfiker 1984:118–122; also Hilfiker 1985). Although the author's intent was to challenge the profession to create ways physicians could meaningfully address their mistakes, the response of my colleagues who read the journal was not particularly favorable. They focused on the acts of "incompetence" and questionable practices that led to patient harm, and found that the confessional style sentimentalized rather than assumed responsibility for these errors. Introducing a mode of discourse normally confined to private conversations into a public, albeit professional, context took great courage; it also revealed the contexts in which various types of discourse on competence are culturally valued or discouraged by the profession.

Published in Britain, *A Savage Enquiry* (Savage 1986) is an excellent example of the reflective repertoire transferred to public writing. Dr. Wendy Savage, a British consultant in obstetrics, details her legal and ideological struggle with male obstetrical consultants who sought to have her privileges suspended for practicing "incompetently." Savage became the center of a national furor when her privileges were suspended in 1985; the suspension was perceived by Savage, her patients, and her supporters as part of the larger battle over who controls childbirth—patients or physicians. Savage argued that the challenge to her obstetrical competence was but a mask for an ideological and gendered battle over the philosophy of birthing and over who is authorized to set standards of obstetrical practice.[18]

This typology of repertoires on medical competence not only highlights the internal stratification and diverse voices within the medical profession but also focuses the analysis on the different ways cultural authority over the production and meaning of professional competence is maintained. Examples of these repertoires of discourse on competence weave through each of the three ethnographic parts of this book, revealing transformations in relations of power and in the culture of medicine.

The Transformation of the Culture of Competence in Rural Medicine

Contests of Specialty and Gender

Introduction to Part I

Many physicians who came of age during the 1960s and 1970s were powerfully affected by an era that contested the assumptions underlying traditional practices and ideologies, including the conceptions of medical competence established by professional elders. Armed with specialty training in the medical meccas of university hospitals and with visions of new forms of medical practice, some moved to rural areas and there confronted an older generation of general practitioners. This new generation of physicians also participated in the transformations in the gender culture of the country as well. The women's health movement in general, and the natural and home birth movements in particular, reframed what was considered appropriate and competent care for women patients, for "mothers and babies." The practice of obstetrics became a domain of innovation and reform as women demanded alternatives, and physicians—both male and female—and midwives responded. Because many of the new physicians were women, they and the midwives brought their own expectations and experiences of giving birth to their medical work. Conflicts over practice styles and competence were thus at times played out as conflicts between men and women practitioners, heightening the gendered character of competence debates.

In this section, the meaning of medical competence in the worlds of practicing clinicians is considered through the lens of an ethnographic story. The story is about the evolution of relationships among obstetrical providers and transformations in obstetrical practice in one rural town in California, which I call "Coast Community," over the course of a decade. The ethnography begins with historical changes in medical practice in rural communities in the region and illustrates how the language of competence became the discourse through which new specialists and residency-trained family physicians challenged older general practitioners, established alternative forms of medical practice, and promoted new criteria of medical competence. Although, in Coast Community, all branches of medical practice experienced these challenges and transformations, the practice of obstetrics became a focus for innovation, heavily influenced by "gendered ways of knowing and doing" and by a professional rethinking of approaches to obstetrical care. It also became an arena for professional and public discussion and contests about medical competence. The story culminates in a crisis of competence which was precipitated by a malpractice suit and by gender and specialty conflicts. Although the details of this ethnographic account are particular to the medical communities in the region I studied, the story is familiar to physicians and patients throughout rural America today. I conclude this section with an analysis of national parallels to the local ethnography and the impact of the national crisis in malpractice and obstetrical care on the specialties of obstetrics and family medicine. The research texts for the national story are drawn from the medical specialty literatures of the period.

The Ethnographic Setting

The research on rural medicine took place over a period of eight years.[1] Intensive ethnographies of medical practice and medical politics in three rural regional communities in Northern California, from 1981 to 1983, were complemented by briefer studies of several other medical communities. Coast Community became our primary research site, and we revisited the area for periods of research in 1985 and 1987 and followed events "at a distance" into the 1990s. Fieldwork included not only living and working in the region but focused interviews with physicians, midwives, nurse practitioners, patients, and community members involved in the community's medical politics as we explored the historical changes and current transformations of rural medicine and primary care. The ethnographic texts I drew on for chapters 2–4 come primarily from this research in Coast Community, although my analysis is informed by research from the other regions that have similar stories to tell.

Coast Community, a district hospital catchment area, had acquired a new public district hospital (licensed for fifty-one beds) in the 1970s to replace older privately owned institutions. The hospital was located in the region's administrative center, a lumber and fishing town with a population of approximately 5,000, but most of the district's population of 50,000 lived in other small towns and in sparsely populated rural environs, on ranches, small farms, and homesteads. Three struggling industries—commercial fishing, lumbering, and tourism—were the economic mainstays of the area, but much employment was seasonal, and during the initial years of the study, unemployment ranged between 9 and 11 percent and again became a very significant problem at the beginning of the 1990s as the lumbering and fishing industries began to collapse. The longitudinal nature of the field research has influenced how I view the contemporary transformation of medical culture in this part of rural North America.

Repertoires of Competence Discourse

The discursive repertoires on medical competence structured many of the changes in the culture of rural medicine. As the ethnographic story unfolds, these discourses flourish, at times mislabeling or masking the turf battles between generalists and specialists, the contests over philosophies and practices in obstetrical care, and the deeply gendered conflicts over medical knowledge and practice hierarchies. Competence and risk became dominant themes as the malpractice and obstetrical crises evolved at both local and national levels. And as the new physicians brought to public awareness what typically had been regarded as suitable only for professional consumption, they often breached boundaries of traditional professionalism that had been protective of traditional medical hierarchies and hegemony and challenged the "conspiracy of silence." This is the story I examine in the following pages.

CHAPTER TWO

The Challenge to
Local Medicine

The practice of medicine in American rural communities was an entrepreneurial endeavor throughout much of the
twentieth century. In rural communities of northern California, successfully staffed hospitals at midcentury were often owned by physician-
entrepreneurs who invested both professionally and financially in their
communities. Centers of urban medicine, both university and corporate, were but marginally related to most of these institutions. Medical
education and state licensure, as well as state medical societies and
hospital accreditation commissions, fostered certain standards of competence and care, yet rural medicine was the domain of the general
practitioner, and physician competence was defined through the practice and standards of generalist colleagues. These physicians, at times
referred to as "local medical docs," possessed varied training, from extensive rotating internships in medicine and surgery and partial residencies to a single year of basic internship in medicine. Well into midcentury, physicians such as these set local standards of competence and
care and adjusted their university knowledge to the context of local
practice.[1]

The decade of the 1970s witnessed the final phasing out of rural
hospitals owned by local physicians in northern California. Some communities in the rural north continued to be served by county-owned
hospitals; these tended to be erratically staffed and isolated institutions with little relationship to centers of medical education and high-
technology medicine. Other communities built new hospitals under

district governance, financed initially with federal and state funds, and managed by public district boards or by private management corporations that specialized in rural hospitals, such as Eskaton and Humanex. These new institutions, with new governance and economic agendas, sought to recruit residency-trained physicians to their medical staffs— specialists in pediatrics, medicine (cardiology), surgery (orthopedics and general surgery), and obstetrics. The new specialists were expected to enhance revenues as well as to "update" services.

New hospitals precipitated the challenge of the specialists to rural medicine. They also became arenas where turf battles and conflicts over standards of practice and medical competence were played out. Organizational changes and specialist review of privileges pitted the "old docs," often generalists, against the "new docs," often specialists recruited by the new hospital administrators. In the experience of many generalists who had previously dominated the medical traditions in their community hospitals and who considered themselves the arbiters of local medical competence, the new hospitals became the theater of their demise, where their expertise, knowledge, and experience were challenged by those who carried the authoritative word from centers of university and corporate medicine on what constituted medical competence.

Rural hospitals have traditionally been notorious as the site of fierce medical turf battles, certainly long before the arrival of specialists.[2] But the introduction of specialty medicine colored rivalries between physicians with an unprecedented aura of gravity and seriousness. Questioning the competence of one's colleagues carried far more weight when representatives of standards of practice produced at the "centers" of medical learning were the judges who recommended proctoring or restriction of privileges. The transition to dominance by specialists within rural medical communities was not necessarily unidirectional nor immediate; in some communities the process would go on for several decades.

During the decades of the 1970s and 1980s, the practice of medicine and the delivery of hospital-based care began to undergo a transformation—a transformation that varied in its rapidity depending on the attractiveness of a rural community and to some extent on the population density of a region. Although I characterize this transformation of the late twentieth century as "the challenge of the specialists" to rural medicine, it is also a story of a generational change in the training of physicians and reflects a radical change in economic interests and professional investment in community hospital medicine.

It is a story in progress, filled with intermittent fits and starts and often poor medical service for some communities, while other communities have experienced extraordinary developments in the quality, complexity, costliness, and diversification of medical and hospital services. In the decade of the 1990s, it has also become a story of financial distress for many community hospitals and a period of reconfiguration of medical practices, as physicians, even "specialists," have been compelled to adapt to new economic and organizational pressures as providers of medical care.[3] Most particularly, as I analyze this period, it is a story about what competence means to community physicians and how local "discourses on physician competence" were generated and shaped by structural changes in the organization and practice of medicine in rural America in the 1980s.

Specialty Boundaries and Competence Talk

Even by 1980, when my husband and I first began our study of primary care in rural northern California, not all communities could boast the presence of board certified internists or surgeons. However, in those communities where board certified specialists had recently joined medical staffs of local hospitals, generalist physicians were often professionally embattled. In response to what I thought was a clichéd question—What was most stressful about being a rural physician?—a former chief of staff at a local hospital vociferously complained that the most stressful thing about practicing medicine was the new doctors in town. Curiously, the new doctors had been recruited by the hospital administration after the hospital itself had been transferred from county control to management by a private corporation. The physician told me what distressed him and how relationships with other physicians had changed since he first came to town:

The new doctors who have recently arrived in this town are all specialists, although the internists and pediatricians call themselves family practitioners. Practicing medicine here used to be great. You were on your own here. There was something new all the time; it is more challenging than academia [he had previously taught anatomy in a large prestigious medical school in another state]. When I first arrived here, we were all GPs, with two surgeons. We'd all help each other out. Everyone was helpful and supportive. Now with these new internists, everyone is out for himself. It is not the same. The first internists—I was instrumental in bringing them here—were fantastic. If you had a problem or thought you were missing something, they'd explain it to you. But these guys—we could learn so much from these guys—but these guys are trying to drive all the old guys out.

He continued, shaking his head:

I don't know why this move to revoke hospital privileges, to proctor us. I don't know what it is, why this has happened. We've asked, but they won't tell us. I would like to know what it is. When I first came to this town, I used to do things I wouldn't do now, what with this malpractice thing. But I never got into any trouble; everything I did came out all right. If you had trouble, you'd get a consult [from a larger town about thirty minutes distant or a medical center one hour and fifteen minutes by car]. Well today . . . these internists present a challenge to my own sense of competence. They are always taking pot shots. But there are a lot of things they can't do that I can, such as setting small fractures. That's the unpleasant thing. We welcomed those guys in and as far as we knew, we were going to be a great working group here.

Interphysician rivalry and conflict within medical communities is amazingly common in rural America, in spite of professional norms and at times "conspiracies of silence."[4] The past two decades have witnessed an unprecedented influx of residency-trained physicians into previously underserved areas (Light 1988; Schwartz 1989; Williams et al. 1983). This change in the profile and density of physicians has frequently jostled professional relationships and introduced a wider potential for questioning the performance of physicians. Advances in biomedicine that have contributed to the flux in specific content of medical expertise, technical competence, and standards of clinical practice provide powerful content to expressions of conflict and turf battles. Thus, it was not surprising that in communities such as those we studied, cleavages emerged between the "old docs" who had been the primary providers of care and the more recently and highly trained "new docs."

The dismay expressed by the rural physician, who until recently had been chief of the medical staff, elected by a community of his peers, highlights the relationship between the structural and demographic changes in the organization of rural medicine. These structural changes introduced a new hierarchy into the community of rural physicians, one that places some physicians above others in terms of "training" and "certification" and "authorized knowledge." Rivalry among physicians was articulated in talk about the competence of other doctors. Unlike the discourse earlier in the century, however, this competence discourse carried authority from the hierarchy of expertise and was rife among physicians in all the rural medical communities we visited. The former chief of staff's comments illustrate the intense personal feelings that are aroused by the expression of that rivalry through disparaging the competence of "the old guys."

Some general practitioners made peace with the new specialists; others were deeply wounded, withdrew from practice, or left to practice medicine elsewhere. Some who weathered the influx of specialists countered the questioning of their own competence with arguments that they had greater breadth of knowledge and years of experience. In their view, new specialists often lacked breadth of knowledge and experience and failed to provide appropriate consulting services. Instead of following the old norm of "availability" and "affability," some new physicians were accused of being intermittently unavailable and hostile to their generalist colleagues. This stance appears to be more common when specialists enter into competition with generalists for primary care patients. One older general practitioner who was board certified in family medicine and highly regarded by many of his colleagues for his surgical skills and general medical competence and by others for "knowing his limitations" expressed bitterness at the new order. He remarked: "The specialists here set themselves up as God. For them, nobody else knows a damn thing! They stick together, no matter what." He also suggested that some specialists were overly narrow, lacking knowledge about the history and practice of medicine in the isolated region where he had practiced for a generation.

Obstetrical practice in particular is a lightning rod for specialist-generalist conflict. Throughout most of the twentieth century, general practitioners and in some areas lay midwives were the primary caretakers of rural women through labor and delivery. When the specialty of obstetrics-gynecology began to produce physicians who chose to practice in rural areas and when the American College of Obstetrics and Gynecology sought to control and regulate obstetrical practice by all physicians, conflicts proliferated, and debates about standards of practice, experience and knowledge, and obstetrical competence of nonspecialists escalated.[5]

A Case of Specialists versus Generalists: Redefining Competence and Care in Obstetrics at Coast Hospital

In 1972, hospital care in Coast Community was transferred from two physician-owned and -managed hospitals to a newly constructed fifty-one-bed district hospital. The new hospital had extraordinary community support and an elected board that included many of the community's most prominent citizens. The more prestigious of the former private hospitals, a large redwood structure with enormous windows and high vaulted ceilings, had been built early in the century. Although the physicians who owned and staffed the institution had exceptional reputations embellished by stories of cure and care of victims of lumbering accidents in the woods and terrible motor vehicle catastrophes (as Hopkins and Stanford graduates, they embodied competent and aggressive medicine), the very antiquity of the institution harked back to an era of medical practice the community felt it had largely outgrown. The new hospital, built with the assistance of federal Hill-Burton funds, was to become a drawing card for new physicians with residency training. It was to bring the area and its health care into the late twentieth century.

In the early years of the 1970s, there was high community enthusiasm for the expansion of medical care and the perception of a bright future for the development of physician and hospital services. Many felt that the care would come to match at least in quality if not quantity that available in two larger medical centers two hours distant. This was an era before the full onslaught of financial difficulties for hospitals and patients, before DRGs ("diagnostic related groups"), MIAs (medically indigent adults), and the creation of the state's financial Medi-Cal "czar" in an effort to bring medical costs under control and to rationalize payment systems to hospitals and doctors. Community physicians, in particular the few internists and surgeons, and the lay members of the new hospital board, aggressively recruited newly graduated specialists who could keep patients in the community and thus bring financial health to their new institution. Obstetricians, internists, orthopedic surgeons, and pediatricians were encouraged to practice in the area with the enticement that not only would they be able to live in an exquisitely beautiful place but the hospital facilities and practice arrangements offered would be up-to-date, even though far from metropolitan medical centers.

Prior to the arrival of board certified obstetricians in 1973 and 1975, the authorized practice of obstetrics on the coast was largely the domain of general practitioners. Assistance for Caesarean sections and surgical procedures was provided by general surgeons. Standards of practice were adjusted to local contingencies; cases were generally managed without anesthesia, given that there were not sufficient nurse-anesthetists to cover all births. Lay midwifery, especially among recent counterculture migrants to the area, had some popularity; as elsewhere in the state, home births and lay midwifery began to flourish with support from the women's health and natural birthing movements. But physician practice of obstetrics was monitored and reviewed within local contexts and from the perspective of local knowledge and experience. General practitioners of long standing in the community as well as those with a somewhat itinerant background (who worked in the community for but a few years before moving on) shared obstetrical work with obstetrician-consultants in the county seat, approximately two hours away.

Within the first year of the new district hospital's opening, the authorized practice of obstetrics by general practitioners and the local standards of care were suddenly challenged by the arrival of a young board certified obstetrician/gynecologist. To many older general practitioners, his arrival proved threatening, for he brought surveillance, monitoring, and a new professional hierarchy of specialist and generalist. The domain of authorized obstetrical practice was to be challenged by a physician who embodied the authority of university and specialty medicine, who had the *right* to redefine the meaning of competence in obstetrical practice.

As the only board certified obstetrician in the medical community, this new physician, who wore Birkenstocks and sported a shaggy, hippy-style beard, became chief of obstetrics for the hospital. Despite his counterculture appearance and somewhat unconventional practice arrangements (he held office hours only two to three days per week), his training at a prestigious medical school and residency gave him excellent professional credentials, impossible to challenge. Encouraged to establish a practice in the area by the few physicians who were also residency-trained "specialists," he was viewed by many general practitioners with dismay and suspicion. What had been the turf of the general practitioner was suddenly opened to specialist scrutiny and to the restructuring of the boundaries of legitimized practice.

Reflecting on the state of general medical and obstetrical practice at the time of his arrival, the obstetrician articulated themes common to encounters between the specialty-trained younger physicians and the older general practitioners who had provided medical care for many decades to rural America. He told me:

The reputation for obstetrical care here was not good. The basic medical reputation of the whole region was not good. If you got ill—you left—quickly. And you can see from some of the practitioners of that time and the facilities that it was a well-deserved reputation; probably a reputation of a lot of small rural areas, that had physicians who were trained a good while ago, [who] were overburdened, overworked, didn't have a chance for continuing education, didn't have facilities, and were seeing many patients a day. They handed out antibiotics right and left, really not taking or not having the time for diagnosis, maybe being a little burned out. . . . If you see forty patients a day, there is no way you can give them an exam. And beyond that, they [doctors] get real tired. So it's medicine from the doorway.

He contrasted his own position, enhanced with the power of his specialty, with his perception of the rural general practitioners:

I was the first OB/GYN to come up, which means . . . that I was the expert and could do what I wanted. I wasn't coming into a situation with established interests, with many docs who did things in a certain way. . . .

You see, I practiced a whole different type of medicine. I had been through a fairly good residency with the luxury of being a specialist and having time, putting aside the time to see patients.

As the new chief of obstetrics, he took the opportunity to start a review of charts "just to get a feeling for what was going on," and was "amazed" to find a number of cases of seriously neglected labors and failures to give appropriate medications for Rh negative cases or proper levels of oxytocin/pitocin in difficult labors. He evaluated much of local obstetrical practice as "just really poor care under any circumstances. Almost no records, little in the way of notes." And his assumption that there were *no established interests* in how obstetrics was practiced allowed him to wipe the slate clean of the generalists' traditional approach to obstetrics. It also underscored the power of specialty knowledge and the hierarchy of medicine, even when practiced at the periphery.

REDEFINING OBSTETRICAL COMPETENCE

Redefining competence in the context of small rural hospitals occurs not only in interactions between specialist and generalist but also through monitoring of medical records. It is through review of records that practice is surveyed, that the power of a specialty is exercised, that the boundaries of practice can be circumscribed and privileges revoked. As the new obstetrician embarked on his mission to reform obstetrical practice, the issue of the state of physician case records repeatedly surfaced.

Two incidents of neglected labor occurred shortly after the obstetrician's initial chart review, which led him to identify general practitioners whom he viewed to be of marginal competence. In a case of a woman who had been in arrested labor for over thirty-six hours, the obstetrician intervened in a most unconventional manner.

I happened to pass him [the attending physician] in the hall and asked him how she was doing. "Oh, everything's fine." "If you have any problems, give me a call." I found that overnight he had given her some pitocin, it stimulated [labor], started, stopped, but he hadn't gotten X rays. . . . She had now been, for a day and a half, unchanged and in labor. At that point, and I hadn't been asked for a consultation, . . . I did something [for which] I could have gotten into legal trouble. But as chief of OB, I took over the patient's care. I got X rays which showed a contracted pelvis. We did a C section quickly, we got a very bad baby, a depressed baby. . . . [The attending physician] never said a whole lot, but one of his friends, a physician in the area, screamed and threatened lawsuit. "We're going to sue your ass"—that kind of thing.

Threats of suit ensued, but the OB chief discovered that he had the legal prerogative to intervene because of his position as chief. He suspended the attending physician's obstetrical privileges, pending investigation of the case. In the second case, another general practitioner was accused of neglecting patients in secondary arrests of labor and of failure to fill out obstetrical records. His obstetrical privileges were temporarily suspended by the OB chief, who was again threatened with legal action. Yet the doctor who was then chief of the medical staff revoked the physician's total hospital privileges within several weeks of the suspension of obstetrical privileges, again because of failure to fill out records, a failure that carried an automatic suspension.

Physicians familiar with the history of this medical community exclaimed that the young obstetrician was aggressively engaged in actions to curtail the privileges of the older general practitioners, that his motivation was to control and dominate the practice of obstetrics on the coast, that his mode of "consultation" and contesting the competence of the older GPs was peculiarly unconventional. Nevertheless, these events led to a complete review of obstetrical privileges, largely with the support of the new hospital's medical staff. Physicians without specialty training who had been performing surgical obstetrical procedures "because no one else was available" lost their privileges. Others whose charts indicated neglected labor and inappropriate patient care had even minimum obstetrical privileges (uncomplicated vaginal deliveries) revoked or temporarily suspended; this was in the traditionally least contested domain of the general practitioners. In addition to the review of obstetrical privileges, the obstetrician in conjunction with others on the new hospital's medical staff began to introduce rules and regulations for all hospital privileges, instituting the concept of *minimum privileges* and initial proctoring. Over the course of three years, from 1973 to 1976, what had been a rather open and quite local system of authorization of practice and of competence began to be revised. Authority to practice, the recognition and meaning of competence, began to be legitimized not through local needs and standards but through specialty medicine, produced and defined at university and metropolitan medical centers.

The consequence of this redefinition of competence led the older general practitioners to abandon the practice of obstetrics. The most established local general practitioner had earlier begun to withdraw from obstetrics to practice primary care medicine, and although he continued to deliver babies for his friends for approximately one year, he was little touched by the changes introduced by the young specialist. Highly integrated into the local community of physicians and surgeons, and deeply committed to the town, the increasingly older profile of his patient panel reflected the decades of his service to the area but also led him to change the complexion of his medical practice. He became board certified in family practice and gave up obstetrics willingly. By contrast, other physicians were more deeply affected, leaving the community altogether to practice medicine elsewhere. One physician committed suicide, shortly after challenges to his competence and care of patients.

The personal consequences of challenges to one's professional competence can only be surmised for those no longer in the community, but the case of the physician who committed suicide poignantly suggests the potential magnitude of such a redefinition. It also suggests the rapidity with which a professional life can spiral out of control when competence is questioned. According to those who knew him, this physician was a quiet man, approximately fifty years old, when the obstetrician suspended his privileges for failure to give *rogam* (an Rh negative medication) and for neglected delayed labors. Although scheduled to appear before the medical staff to review his case management, he refused to attend. His loss of hospital privileges did not initially deter him from continuing to see obstetrics patients in an office-based practice. Several patients who were told they could not be delivered by their physician found their way to the obstetrician's care, without appropriate referral, when ready to give birth. The obstetrician recalled the case with some sadness.

I reported him because of abandonment of patients. I don't know what came of that, not too much. He was subsequently reported [by others] and investigated and cleared for prescribing medicines without due exam. He had been reported a couple of times and was cleared and was under investigation again when he committed suicide.

Obstetrical care became the domain of the community's new physicians: the obstetrician/gynecologist specialists, who numbered three by 1976, were at the top of the hierarchy, followed by family medicine physicians, certified midwives, young generalists, and lay midwives. Many physicians had itinerant practices; they remained in the community for brief periods and often left to seek additional training. These newcomers to the medical community "consulted" the specialists "appropriately," thus recognizing the hierarchy of specialist and generalist and the obstetrician's right to define the boundaries of obstetrical competence. In contrast to the older GPs who sought to challenge the legitimacy of the specialists' right to authorize competence, through threat of legal action and accusations of limited availability, the new physicians and midwives sought other forms of relationships with the new consultants.

REDEFINING OBSTETRICAL CARE

The reconfiguration of specialist-generalist relationships and the redefinition of what constituted obstetrical competence in the local context was only the beginning of the transformation of obstetrical practice in Coast Community which grew out of the importation of knowledge and standards of university and metropolitan obstetrics. This "medicine of the center" was embodied in the obstetrical specialist and manifested in his professional mission to control, shape, and authorize the practice of obstetrics within his community. However, this mission extended beyond the bounds of the district hospital's medical community. The chief of obstetrics, in conjunction with his partners, began a process that led to the establishment of a family-centered birthing and maternity care program, the first of its kind in the country. The "mission" to reform the practice of birthing brought precisely those struggles which were at the heart of university and metropolitan obstetrics into the rural periphery. And it was at the periphery of university medicine that the revolution in hospital obstetrical care was successfully launched.

In 1973, the vision of family-centered maternity care for all patients was revolutionary for obstetricians, although by no means for large segments of the population. Lay midwives had been creating alternative birthing experiences through providing home births, and family physicians had been lobbying for alternative settings for hospital births with fathers present at delivery. In fact, throughout the state, the home birth movement flourished during the decade of the 1970s, but it occurred largely at the margins of officially authorized medicine and outside the purview of the profession of obstetrics.

In 1972, home births in the remote regions of the Coast hospital district and among members of the counterculture occurred at approximately three or four per month. A limited number of young family physicians participated in the home-birthing movement, delivering babies or offering medical backup to lay midwives. A modified form of natural childbirth in traditional local hospital deliveries had also been encouraged by the older general practitioners, who because of limited resources (only one nurse-anesthetist, who could not be present at all births) rarely used the anesthesia of "metropolitan" obstetrics—spinals, epidurals, caudals. In addition, one family physician who had practiced briefly in the area before moving elsewhere had allowed fathers in the hospital's delivery room. Thus the nonmedical community's expectations provided friendly ground for the introduction of childbirth education and the acceptance of the obstetrician's lead in low intervention and innovative hospital birthing practices.

The community's new obstetricians provided consultant backup for home births attended by lay midwives and family physicians. They did not, however, participate in home births themselves. Instead they developed a family-centered and hospital-based maternity care program that eventually symbolized an assertion of specialty control over the local alternative birthing movement. Shortly after the establishment of the alternative family birthing center under the obstetricians' guidance, home births declined to fewer than one per month.

GOING PUBLIC

Initial developments in reforming birthing practices in the district hospital led to a certain amount of turmoil and friction among the hospital nursing staff, the administrator, the elected board, and the specialists. As recounted by the physician who was chief of obstetrics at the time, sheer "force" and more "vinegar than honey" were used to bring about changes. Successive appeals to a largely supportive public, the hospital board, and the state's regulatory health boards were among the strategies employed by the specialists, who continued to be viewed by many in the traditional health care community as "radicals" or "hippies" with extreme ideas. One partner recalled the very lengthy "battles" to bring about reforms. However, the lengthy battles occurred over a strikingly short period of three years.

The changes in routine birthing practices began innocuously enough, and fathers were "encouraged" whether or not they had had childbirth training to be present at the birth. The presence of fathers in the delivery room evolved as routine practice. Active opposition from nursing administration led to additional disputes over the attendance at births of "partners" and other family members, including children. A series of incidents, including one in which a woman wished her six-year-old to be present at the birth of her new sibling, led to a further revolution in defining who could be present at a birth. The obstetrician responsible, in recalling how it became a cause celebre, related the following:

She was planning on delivering at home; she was uncomfortable with delivering at home, but she had a six-year-old daughter who was very much a part of the whole process, attending all the classes with her. And her daughter wanted to be at the birth and that was impossible at the hospital, because no kids under twelve were allowed in the hospital, much less at the birth. I checked into this to see if this was the law. And not only was it not the law that kids couldn't be at the birth, there was no law about it one way or another. There are many things in bureaucratic institutions that are considered law, but when you look into it, it's not law, it's just been done that way for so many years that everyone considers it law. But the law had changed the previous year, that young kids couldn't be present in hospitals—they could. I contacted the Department of Health and got an OK to have this kid at the birth. It was the first child in the States present at an in-hospital birth. It became a cause celebre at the time and was written up in the [national press]. And this was the first real birthing center.

In this case, as in many others, the chief of obstetrics presented his arguments to change policy to the public. In seeking special "dispensation" for this patient's child, he brought birthing out of the home and into the hospital and thus under the specialist's control. Appealing to the new state law that allowed children to be present without restriction in hospital settings, albeit at family discretion, he overrode the protests of the hospital administrator and traditional nursing staff and sought support for this action from the community board as well as from the state. With this crack in the traditional routine of practice, the OB chief requested approval of a pilot project in family-centered maternity care. The new program would allow fathers to assist in delivery if they wished, children would be welcome, and nurses trained in obstetrics would be on call, guiding patients through labor and into delivery.

Remarkably, the obstetricians' battle to change the birthing routine of the hospital coincided with a battle over therapeutic abortions. As in many American communities, therapeutic abortions were hotly contested, and certain hospital administrators, including nursing administrators, resisted hiring not only nurses who were specialists in obstetrics but also nurses who would be willing to care for patients who had undergone therapeutic abortions. The contest between the obstetricians and the hospital administration came to a head when a patient who was scheduled for a therapeutic abortion was visited in her room by the hospital administrator, who tried to convince her not to undergo the procedure. The incident was publicized in the local press by the obstetricians and taken to the board; the nursing and hospital administrators were fired and replaced by individuals more amenable to the obstetricians' project. The change in personnel was highly significant, and allowed the next phase of the reform to proceed—the hiring of specialist OB nurses—and curiously, the feminization of routine hospital birthing care.

The concurrent construction of a birthing room out of two small labor rooms occurred in response not only to the forcefulness of the specialists in realizing their project goals but also to the hospital's sensitivity to desires of the public. They also recognized the skill with which the obstetricians mobilized community support and interest. The new birthing room and new birthing "beds," constructed of local Madrone wood by a famous local woodworker, symbolized the *local* revolution in the meaning of "care" in obstetrics.

The family-centered birthing pilot project that had been approved by the state's infant health unit included a prospective and retrospective study of infection rates, complications, and outcomes. After a review of the findings, in which no significant difference in infection rates was found (in fact they appeared to be lower), the project was declared a success two and one-half years after its inauguration. Thus, the Coast hospital possessed *the first official family-centered maternity care program in the country.* It was visited by obstetricians from university hospitals who sought to pattern their new programs after this rural innovation.

The innovation in birthing practices in this community did not occur in an ideological vacuum, but rather represented one vanguard in obstetrics. The obstetricians were influenced not only by their training in Lamaze units, rather unique experiences for university obstetrics residencies in 1970, but also by the worldwide childbirth movement of which some obstetricians were a part. Clearly the OB chief's participation in the International Childbirth Education Association fueled his enthusiasm for these reforms, and he recollected:

I started out with a larger purpose in mind [changing birthing practices in obstetrics] and quickly got down to just our very local thing. When I was on the board of the ICEA, I spoke at lots of conferences. Once the program got settled here and other things got really rolling, I haven't done that really at all. Local things—starting to realize that is all I could manage. And yet, it is still a battle to be fought.

Another obstetrician recounted how he had worked to include fathers in delivery both during his residency training and later when he was in the public health service. "I would say, do you want to see your baby being born? Come on in to the delivery room! We don't have an alternative birthing center here—this is it!"

The struggle to overcome traditional bureaucratic and administrative barriers to authorize routine alternative birthing practices and to reform the meaning of obstetrical care was not only to improve the experience of mothers, babies, and families, but was for the obstetricians' enjoyment as well. In recollecting the efforts to reform the routine practice of birthing on the Coast, an obstetrician commented:

As far as all the efforts we put into this community, it was self-serving; it was for *us,* too. *We* wanted to work in [this] kind of environment, . . . we wanted to do natural childbirth, and we wanted to have the birthing situation we created. So it wasn't totally altruistic. But we certainly had to fight for it too.

Despite this revolution at the periphery, even with its influence on the birthing practices at centers of university obstetrics in the region, these now rural-based obstetrical specialists acknowledged the contrary and dominant modes in the practice of university obstetrics. High-risk patients and pathological and risk-oriented obstetrics are the norm of the training context; nonintervention, low-risk obstetrical practice remains largely a marginal activity. In commenting on a noted university program, one of the obstetricians remarked that few university physicians practice in the alternative birthing centers of their own departments. This perception foreshadowed a similar change in the configuration of practice and in the standards of care and competence for low-risk obstetrics at Coast hospital.

The Feminization of Obstetrical Care and Competence

The hiring of nurses who were specialists in obstetrics brought a level of nursing competence to labor and delivery practices previously unseen in this medical community. As these women guided patients through the course of labor and delivery, they began the process of the feminization of low-risk obstetrical *care* at Coast hospital and contributed in a highly visible manner to the success of the hospital's family-centered maternity care. By the late 1970s, the obstetricians also began to incorporate midwives into their own practice, and through that incorporation authorized a feminine form of competence in hospital obstetrics. Birthing, from labor through delivery and postnatal care, could be carried out entirely by a female staff. Competence and hierarchy were assured by the specialists' arrangements with the midwives, who were employed *by* them, and with the OB nurses, who were employed *for* them by the hospital administration.

Inadvertently, the move to incorporate OB nurses and certified nurse-midwives into hospital-oriented obstetrical care also sowed the seeds for a resurgence of home births in the region. As home births increased, the obstetricians willingly provided consultant backup for the home births attended by "their" midwives and OB nurses.

A lay midwife and former patient who worked for the obstetricians for three years, doing postnatal home visits, mused on her perception of changes that led to the feminization of care. Women professionals soon came to mediate and shape the relationship between obstetrics patients and their male obstetricians.

These physicians would take criticism very much to heart. "You don't spend time with people afterward" . . . "You just come in," et cetera. And they hired midwives to replace that aspect of what they did, and they hired me. I remember the first week I started work . . . and [one of the OBs] asked me, "How do you like your new job?" "Oh—I really enjoy it. I can see now why you needed somebody to do this, why people ask me questions they would never ask you." And he said, "Well, what would they ask you they wouldn't ask me?" I said to him, "You tell me the last time you sat down with a new mother and listened for twenty minutes to every time the baby fed for three days, feeding by feeding." He said, "Oh well, I haven't done that . . . I guess,

seeing them—my life doesn't have the time to do that, I do other things."
But it was so much as though he was saying, "I don't do that, do I? I do tech
and I've moved into specialization—which is good, I like that, but I've also
cut off that kind of interaction."

The midwives who joined the obstetricians' practice brought their
own particularly female experiences to their interaction with patients.
And although formal training was of critical importance, it was the
personal and female birthing experiences that attracted many women
to rethink the practice of birthing. Indeed, these experiences came to
inform much of their practice and their mode of caring.

A nurse-midwife who had joined the obstetricians' practice in the
late 1970s recounted the path that brought her to midwifery.

I had done five years of newborn intensive care nursing, a year of labor and
delivery nursing, a year of public health nursing, specializing in maternal
and infant health. But what really changed things for me—from being into
the high tech—newborn intensive care is very crazy—*I had a baby. And my
own birth was pretty horrendous,* really, and I realized that for the majority of
women who were having births, this was what it was like. *And I was appalled!*

Being appalled led her to attend a meeting of people interested in trying to change the practice of hospital obstetrics in the state, and her
passion for "mothers and babies" proved to be a major resource for
the region's new birthing consumer movement.

There were a number of people who had home births and were interested in
having home births—and when they found out that there was a registered
nurse that was sympathetic *and* experienced in taking care of sick babies, I was
invited to my first home birth. [By] word of mouth, things just progressed.
The last year and a half I was doing seven to ten births a month in [Sacra-
mento] and eight surrounding counties. . . . I was trucking. . . . And then the
opportunity came to go to school—so I went.

After one year of training in midwifery, in the state's first program that
led to licensure, she chose to join the obstetricians' practice, where
the "radical" innovation in hospital birthing was successfully instituted,
the battle fought, and midwifery privileges for hospital deliveries approved. In commenting on why she did not return to her home city
to work with a "very sweet obstetrician," she noted, "I would have
had to be a battering ram for changing things [to gain hospital privi-
leges]. . . . I was battle weary. I just wanted to go somewhere, where I
could *just* practice. . . . I didn't want to change a million people's
minds." Definitely *not* wanting to practice traditional OB, she found

the alternative offered by the Coast hospital to be a "nice compromise between hospital and home." The birthing center she discovered in 1979 was an ideal context in which to continue working for "mothers and babies."

People could have their friends and family with them. They could go home early; they didn't have to be *messed with,* didn't have to have . . . routine things done to them. The doctors were into nurse-midwives, and realized they could benefit from utilizing their services, in more ways than one.

The feminization of obstetrical care received its impetus from numerous sources, some particular to the local context and culture and others more societal in nature. In terms of local context, the obstetricians/gynecologists sought to design an ideal organization of practice for themselves, which would allow for flexibility of coverage and sabbatical leaves. The sabbatical option (three-month leave each year) meant that "we were not necessarily here or around and it was impossible to assure someone that this [particular] doctor would deliver." Yet the obstetricians' definition of good care, also a prevailing ideology in the specialty, that "ideal care for the OB patient is to see one person who delivers you; no question about it," conflicted with this organization of practice. Confronted with competing desires and goals, the specialists resolved the conflict through a radical restructuring of their practices and the introduction of nurse-midwives. At the societal level, the women's health movement was highly influential in obstetrics itself, shaping reforms and changes within obstetrical practice and obstetrical ideology, encouraging the involvement of nurse-midwives in prenatal care, and in the more innovative metropolitan and university programs encouraging nurse-midwives' management of birthing. The culture of the local community fit very well with the obstetricians' goals; the community prided itself on its progressive vision of medical practice and health care, and midwives were viewed as highly desirable and not necessarily revolutionary care providers.

By 1980, the obstetricians' midwives managed the majority of low-risk patients and essentially did "all the normal OB," as one of the obstetricians recalled. The doctors shared call with the midwives, and each partner saw all patients at least once, but the practice had become one in which the attending providers at most births were female nurse-midwives. The obstetricians began to focus on obstetrical and gynecological surgery, infertility technology, and other more specialized activities of their profession.

The Osmosis of "Professional" Knowledge into Home Birthing

Curiously, the introduction of nurses who were specialists in obstetrics and of certified nurse-midwives into the hospital obstetrical community led to a remarkable professionalization of the homebirth movement in the region. Home births "on the side" of official practice were at first tolerated by the obstetricians with benevolence and uncontested consultancies. None of the obstetricians wished to be involved in the practice of home births, and as one midwife told us, "there was plenty of business for everybody." A wide set of choices and alternatives for birthing experiences fit the desires and the *professional ideology* of the obstetricians, as long as the hierarchy of expertise was acknowledged and consultations were made "appropriately and early."

There was an interesting osmosis of professional knowledge into home births, as nurse-midwives introduced the use of external monitors (doptones) and other technologies of hospital births. Technology, albeit low technology, consultant backup, and competence were brought by the certified nurse-midwives to their home-birthing practice. Birth on the margins of the professional domain came under the powerful influence of the obstetrician specialists. These men brought trained women into the community and employed them in their practices; they legitimized and indirectly authorized their alternative practices; they provided consultant backup and specialty expertise and hospital care when needed; and they monitored and reviewed the home-birth activities of their female colleagues. The beneficent dominance by the obstetricians of birthing on the coast gradually came to be challenged only after the arrival of two residency-trained women physicians.

Obstetrical Practice Reconfigured

The attractiveness of the hospital district, the availability of medical resources, and the cultural diversity of the communities in the area drew many new physicians throughout the decade of the 1970s; most had completed residency training and several had done subspecialty fellowships. By 1980, two women, residency trained in family medicine, joined the community of health providers. The first

woman physician established a small family practice and a select obstetrical caseload; she performed only home births. As other nonspecialist providers left the area, she found the demand for her obstetrical
services increased. Eventually, she joined in partnership with a midwife, who had previously worked for the obstetricians as one of their
first obstetrical nurses prior to her midwifery training and licensure.
Their practice was considered by the women of the community to be
highly selective and confined to low-risk home births. It also included
other women health providers in what was characterized by many patients as a feminine if not feminist practice. The practice served the
southern reaches of the hospital district. Initially, the women's practice
was not perceived by the medical community nor by the public as
either an economic or ideological threat to the obstetricians' large and
flourishing practice. The obstetricians were located in the northern-
most town of the hospital district and were close to the hospital and
to the family birthing center.

Within a year after the initial creation of the "feminine" practice, a
second woman family physician moved to the region and joined the
practice as a semi-partner—a colleague who shared office overhead,
call, and backup for obstetrical cases. She brought a flair for children
and a style of practice that was less exclusive than that of her partners.
She too began to practice home births, with the occasional assistance
of the midwife and office staff. Gradually both physicians began to do
some hospital obstetrics, along with their nurse-midwife. Differences
in the style and philosophy of practice led the women to dissolve the
partnership after four years; however, they continued to offer backup
for each other and occasional call coverage. In the minds of the community, even in the minds of their medical colleagues, the two women,
who were extraordinarily different in their medical style, were frequently spoken about as a couple, or interchangeably. As these women's
respective practices grew larger and as they began to cross into the obstetricians' domain, the tensions between the female family physicians
and their nurse-midwife partners and the male specialists intensified,
leading to a simmering "turf battle" that eventually had serious consequences for obstetrics as practiced "on the coast." It was in the context of this turf battle that a crisis of competence was precipitated by a
malpractice suit against the obstetricians.

The presence of women physicians who practiced obstetrics somewhat independently, and some would claim differently, from the male
obstetricians, transformed the specialist-generalist relationship that had

evolved during the decade of the 1970s under the dominance of the obstetricians. Suddenly, obstetrical care was not only carried out by women who were controlled and monitored by the male obstetricians—the definers of what constituted competent as well as caring practice—but was practiced by these new women who were certified and licensed. Their practice was authorized through family medicine residency training or midwifery certification, a competence earned and to some extent granted independently of the obstetricians. Experiences of birthing and pre- and postnatal care were created through an ideology of feminine obstetrical practices. The ideological stance of the women's practices influenced how obstetrical work was carried out. It also affected the professional relationships the women developed with their colleagues, the male specialists.

In a sense, the male obstetricians and the women physicians and midwives introduced new varieties of local practice and local knowledge to obstetrics on the coast in the late 1970s and throughout the decade of the 1980s. However, their projects, which at times appeared to be joint or collegial efforts to improve the quality of obstetrical competence and care for patients—mothers and babies—were also distinguished because of differences in gender and specialty. These differences led to cultural conflicts and distinctions in practice, types of knowledge, and assessment of competence.

CHAPTER THREE

Competence and Care

Cultural Conflicts Embedded in Gender and Specialty

They [the male obstetricians/gynecologists] don't have the same feeling for it, or as a community of women have for other women. Sure there are areas where they know a lot more than we do. And there are areas where you cannot explain [what is known]. It is as if you are talking a different language.

—A midwife

R. believes he's better at doing OB than we are—all across the board. He doesn't begin to understand what people don't get by going to them that they get from us. [He] does not know what it is that we're doing that he's not, that matters, and that's increasingly OK with me.

—A family physician

Those girls are going to get into trouble [with the medical community], doing home deliveries. . . . Of course, that's how we used to practice; low intervention, no pit, no induced labors, some home deliveries.

—A general practitioner

The essence of the practice of medicine gains form from physicians' articulation of what they know and how they know it. Individual practices are informed not only by a physician's formal knowledge but by experiential knowing. The common refrain in medicine—

"in my experience . . ."—has come to be viewed with skepticism, especially since the rise of clinical epidemiology; it remains exalted, however, in the medical teaching cliche "see one, do one, teach one." Knowledge and experience are intimately linked for clinicians.

The reconfiguration of obstetrics on the coast and the feminization of obstetrical practices and care led to a professional and *very public* articulation of a feminine way of knowing, a feminine form of obstetrical knowledge and therefore of obstetrical competence. This public and professional expression held that competence included tacit and experiential knowledge as well as knowledge authorized through formal medical training. And it contributed to the gender distinctions and the intraprofessional discourses that came to characterize this community of obstetrical providers in the decade of the 1980s.

By the early 1980s, gender and specialty coincided almost perfectly. The obstetrician specialists and surgeons were males; the family physicians who offered low-intervention obstetrical care and the midwives were females; all the women had given birth at least once and one had six children. Male family physicians and general practitioners no longer offered routine obstetrical care to the coastal community. This structural configuration provided the cultural grist for the discourse on obstetrical competence, caring, and competition. Distinctions of gender and specialty colored how these physicians and midwives produced and regarded competing forms of knowledge relevant to obstetrical practice.

Bringing passion to medical work is an intermittent experience, particularly in obstetrics. The previous chapter documented the fervor brought by the male specialists to reforming hospital obstetrical care. Passion generated by the sense of carrying the knowledge of the specialist, earned and authorized at university centers of specialty training, fueled the obstetricians' success. An equally purposive and passionate commitment to reforming the experience of birthing and expanding women's choices came to characterize the women's obstetrical practices. Whereas the male obstetricians of Coast Community reformed hospital-based obstetrical care and brought the family-centered alternative birthing unit into being, the women family physicians and "independent" midwives broadened women's choices by offering competent and licensed coverage for home births as well as hospital births. They also created a different type of birthing experience which became the "standard of care" in the eyes of many pregnant women in the community. Whence came the passion, the knowledge infused with affect, which propelled these women toward redesigning and feminizing obstetrical practice?

The Experiential Transformation of Professional Knowledge

When physicians analyze the source of their medical knowledge, they frequently distinguish experiential knowledge from knowledge formally learned in the context of medical training (see Jordan 1989). For the women physicians in practice in Coast Community, home births brought an opportunity to right what they had perceived as the wrongs of their high-risk obstetrical training in hospital-based residencies. The midwives, many of whom had previously worked in traditional high-risk obstetrical nursing, brought their own unique professional training and philosophy of low-intervention birthing to home births and to hospital births, as described in the previous chapter. The women physicians and midwives felt that high-intervention obstetrical practice was altogether too common and inappropriate as the *standard* for obstetrics. In their view, such practice negatively colored the birthing experience for many low-risk women. And when they recalled their own personal experiences with standard obstetrical care, it was frequently with intense negative emotions.

Transformation of the meaning of knowledge often involves reflections on personal experiences. In this case, the women practitioners drew on their own individual births and professionally attended births as sources for redefining what women's birthing experiences should be. The explicit recognition of new meanings attached to previous birthing experiences led these women to redefine the kind of knowledge that was relevant to competent and caring obstetrical practice. Doing home births also allowed for a different kind of knowledge to be learned *through* practice as well as to be employed *in* practice.

PERSONAL EXPERIENCE REINTERPRETED

One of the physicians, who at the time of our interviews was in her early forties, had chosen to establish a practice in this community to escape the pressures of metropolitan medicine and to care for patients in an innovative and more humanistic way. She recalled her initial training in high-risk obstetrics and how she was "appalled" by the style and standard of practice at her residency training hospital. Unable at the time to "trust" her own sense of "appalledness," she neither expressed nor acted on her feelings. She became increasingly uneasy with what passed for standard obstetrical care during the births of her two children. She characterized her first child's birth as "just awful"—laboring alone for many hours in a darkened room—"but passing for an ordinary birth" and interpreted her second pregnancy as an attempt to correct what had gone wrong, "a very common phenomenon when somebody has a terrible first birth." Although continuing obstetrics in training and in her first private practice, she resisted analyzing what she was doing with patients and what her own birthing experiences meant to her, professionally and personally. At the time, she told me she had no sense that her personal experience had been "a disaster for me, no sense of the misery, no sense of the terror. I lived it but didn't apprehend it." Although she discontinued offering obstetrical care shortly after completing residency, she felt unable at the time to formulate *why*, recalling that at the last delivery, "I had a sense of something being terribly wrong. But I didn't say in my own mind at the time—as I was sitting there at the end of the table with the forceps—'something is terribly wrong.' With a knocked-out lady, right."

For this physician, redefining the personal and professional experience of birthing came over the course of several years. Initial insights that developed from leading psychotherapy groups were later fed by her growing awareness of the feminist and alternative literature on birthing. Reading Suzanne Arms's *Immaculate Deception* (1975) led her to reframe her own birthing and obstetrical training experiences. New opportunities to reenter family practice and obstetrics led the physician to channel what had been an inner and unarticulated sense of rage to an outwardly directed passion and a concern to transform the experience of birthing for pregnant women under her care. This new experiential knowledge, infused with a sense of passion, clarified the kind of actions she sought to take, to right the wrongs in the practice of obstetrics. Thus, she made the decision to perform a small number of home births.

I was going to do a few home births. [Why?] Because I was so tired of . . . moaning about the state of the world I wanted to do something. . . . Really I was so sick of my own bile that I never wanted to complain again, I just wanted to make a difference. . . . Most of it came from wanting other women to experience their experience instead of going through what I went through. That's where seventy-five percent came from. Rage. Rage at what happens to women. You see, my personal opinion is that those experiences leave very deep marks that no amount of words can ever erase.

The physician's choice to do home births in her newly established practice was a decision to create an arena in which she could apply insights about the limits of high-risk hospital obstetrical training. Home births would also provide an arena in which knowledge gained through the personal experience of giving birth and attending at births could be acted upon in an effort to create a positive and enjoyable experience for women. After several years of attending home births, first solely and then with partners (a team of women which included another physician, certified nurse-midwives, obstetrical nurses, and lay midwives with specialties in child development and mother-infant bonding), she noted that home births were not only

a major part of what I do . . . it's also a major part of what does me. . . . The process has at least as much impact on me as I have upon it. And in pursuing it with passion, I have been probably transformed, I would say. That is not an exaggeration.

Personal passion, derived from reflective knowledge, led to an evolving ideological stance in the physician's obstetrical work. And it was this stance that quickly attracted other partners and a growing number of patients to her care. The other women who joined the practice came with their own visions of how to alter the birth experience, with their own personal experiences, positive as well as negative, in giving and doing births. The ideological position of the practice, however, remained clear; it emphasized maternal choice and low-intervention birthing. Hospital births, when accepted, were to be managed as similarly as possible to home births, and women were to be protected from arbitrary interventions and decisions. Although a somewhat fluctuating set of women health providers participated in the obstetrical team of midwives, physicians, and birth attendants, and although internal differences over styles of practice occasionally surfaced, what constituted relevant knowledge for obstetrical practice was seldom in dispute.

PROFESSIONAL KNOWLEDGE REINTERPRETED

The women practitioners frequently contrasted knowledge gained in the home-birth context about the natural progression from labor to birthing with the technical medical knowledge of high-risk obstetrics learned in residency training, experiences shaped by hospital standards of care and organizational constraints. They came to use a language of "transformation," "intuition," "qualitative," and "instinctual" to describe experiential knowledge gained through home births. And although competence in obstetrical procedures was certainly considered relevant for home births (and indeed loomed in importance when difficulties arose), the incorporation of experiential knowledge through practice became a major *professional* task and an important way through which the women defined and framed their work. Personal and experiential knowledge was shared, thereby shaping a subcommunity increasingly organized by gender and specialty and with a distinctive intraprofessional discourse on obstetrical competence.

The redefinition of what constituted appropriate knowledge for obstetrical practice continued to emerge through doing home births. One of the physicians related how her considerations had been transformed through doing home births.

I had my background in high-risk obstetrics. Most of the time that was more of a hindrance than a help. I practically learned from scratch [while doing home births]. It was great taking the blinders off. . . . So many of the things that I had noticed in passing before but didn't understand suddenly became much clearer. I can still remember residents in the delivery units where I first trained opening the pit [oxytocin] when the contractions slowed down in second stage, and nobody told me they would always resume. It has been a wonderful paradigm—looking and seeing what is around me rather than looking and having it filtered through what I was taught, therefore not seeing. . . . For years I was around a lot of phenomena that I was taught to observe in a certain way and therefore other information just never got through to me.

The physicians and midwives frequently contrasted their knowledge with that of the obstetricians as being of a different order, that they saw the same phenomena through a different lens. Although the women were generally restrained in their criticisms of the technical competence of the male obstetricians, and in fact often praised the obstetricians as being "very good" and "excellent surgeons" when intervention was called for, when they recollected and analyzed the process of caring for women in labor and birth, the women characterized their own knowledge and very competence as "birth attendants" as being something quite different from that possessed by their male colleagues.

Standards of practice, judgment over arrested labors, decisions on when to bring someone into the hospital, and questions about how

best to approach breech deliveries were all areas of potential and eventually of active dispute with the obstetrical specialists. Controlled and
low-intervention obstetrical care, women's choice, and maternal/family-
infant bonding were foremost among the women practitioners' concerns. The women's approach not only provided their patients with a
different meaning and context to birthing, but the women reframed
the technical and medical activities performed in the course of delivering competent care. Their particular standards of care were directed to
achieving low intervention and high maternal control during birthing.
In turn, the women practitioners frequently felt at a loss to justify
their practice, what they knew to be their best "judgment," to their
male colleagues, the specialists.

Low-intervention approaches to birthing were the preferred norm
throughout the obstetrical community, regardless of practitioner gender, and the obstetricians characterized the normal deliveries in their
practice as "low intervention for low-risk patients." However, the
women still contrasted their approach to that of the men and held that
they favored to a greater degree low technology and natural processes,
and practice determined by women's choice. The women noted that
low intervention neither meant low expertise nor low contact. Indeed,
when describing their practices, they claimed it was the mixture of their
medical expertise as well as the quality and kind of interactions with
patients that made the obstetrical care they gave unique and special.

Discussions of cases of difficult or delightful labors and deliveries
were frequently framed in terms of "energy" exchanged, of the hyp-
notic dimensions of attendance at birthing, of women moving through
arrested labor to realization that they could overcome the arrest because of the very nature of their interactions with their women physicians, midwives, and other birth attendants. The manner through
which energy was conveyed to women in labor is described as moving
women from distressful states of difficult labor toward transition and
successful births.

One case, related by a physician, highlighted what she regarded as a
joyful success.

A woman who was giving birth to her second child had an unexpectedly difficult labor. During the process of pushing, there was meconium staining, and
the physician wanted the woman not to push, to let the next contraction "dry
the baby out" to eliminate problems from meconium. The woman, who was
in the process of "freaking out," responded to the guidance of her birth attendants and stopped pushing, "stopped freaking out in mid-freak," allowing
the contraction to proceed as desired. As her baby was born, the mother

turned to her birth attendants, saying, "oh you guys, oh you guys, thank you." And in the words of the physician: "And she knew *exactly* what she was thanking us for . . . she would not have gotten that combination of expertise and contact. She could have gotten the expertise, maybe, from other people but at the expense of her presence, and from a lay midwife she'd not gotten the expertise. She knew [what we were giving her]; she was wonderful.

In discussing approaches to getting women to progress through the transition phase in labor, a birth attendant from the practice described how she used her personal touch; by lying next to the laboring woman and embracing her, she was able to encourage progression. She recalled: "[Through the] transference of energy, through focusing my concentration on hers" and "without a need to explain what was occurring, the experience of being geared to that phenomenon, experientially, something was exchanged instantly."

For this group of women practitioners, the mixture of obstetrical competence with their unique approach to being with patients led them to distinguish their practice from that of the male specialists. They always took care in these accounts not to tarnish the midwives in the obstetricians' practice. In part, the distinction was one of place and the structure and constraints of place. Hospital births, even in the family-centered unit, were simply more formalized in terms of standards of practice and care than were home births. Furthermore, these women practitioners also attended hospital births, albeit somewhat reluctantly. Even in this setting, efforts were made to color the hospital experience as a home birth experience, through the way the birth attendants and physicians interacted with women in labor. Needless to say, it would be difficult and in many communities considered inappropriate for male physicians to embrace patients as they moved through transition.

"Acts of God": Challenge to Low-Intervention Birthing

Extraordinary clinical events, unforeseen medical catastrophes—"acts of God"—impress physicians and midwives with the limits of medical knowledge and the uncertainty of their art. Neonatal deaths, "bad babies," and other difficulties were rare experiences among the Coast obstetrical practices; yet, the obstetricians, family physicians, and midwives all had occasions that led them to reconsider their obstetrical work. Specialists can use these rare events when they wish to raise questions about a practitioner's competence and expertise or when they seek to circumscribe practice domains. For the clinicians involved, however, such events can lead to painful reflections on uncertainty in medicine and in particular on threats to their own deeply personal sense of competence. These personal responses leave individuals vulnerable to professional criticism. In such a climate, practices emphasizing low intervention and home birthing can be cast into an arena of professional "risk" and birthing choices can be jeopardized.

The following case of the death of an infant exemplifies how an achieved sense of competence is threatened by such an "act of God," and how efforts at repair are undertaken through both reflective and intraprofessional discourse. In the case I describe, the obstetrical specialists did not question the competence of the women physicians and midwives involved, nor did they use this case as a cause celebre to curtail home births. Ironically, it occurred concurrently with other infant deaths that led to a malpractice crisis for the obstetricians and their midwifery colleagues, which was later to have ramifications for the entire obstetrical provider community. However, the case had profound personal meanings for those most closely involved, eventually leading some of the birth attendants to discontinue their obstetrical work.

Several years after the women's home birth practice began to flourish, one of the family practice physicians encountered what she referred to as "the existential issue in medicine." The obstetrical care offered by the physician and her partners was highly sought after, widely known, and respected for low intervention, high quality, and successful home birthing. When one of her patients gave birth to an unexpectedly highly distressed infant who died shortly after birth, the physician was in attendance with two midwives with whom she shared her practice. All three women were stunned. In reflecting on the infant's unexpected death, the physician told me she fought an overwhelming sense of uncertainty and surprise at the baby's death, which led her to review her performance and that of her colleagues.

It just never occurred to me because it has never happened to me, that if I took super good care of someone and was really there, that things wouldn't go well. I am not saying that I haven't had "acts of God" before; I certainly have. But none of them have been fatal. In fact, I would say that on the whole, "acts of God" are a hell of a lot fewer than one would think. A lot of what passes as "acts of God" are people not paying attention at an energy level—which was certainly not true in this case. You cannot imagine the shock,

assuming the baby is fine because the parameters are fine. [It is] totally different from knowing that I have a distressed baby and preparing for the worst,
which I've done before. Knowing a baby is compromised and getting ready
for it—who likes that? But I accept that as part of my work. Thinking that
the baby is normal and having it come out almost dead is just not to be believed. . . . I have never seen that happen. I have seen babies with low fetal
heart tones come out normal. I have never seen a baby with normal fetal heart
tones come out distressed, not even a little.

The physician and her colleagues responded professionally and
emotionally to the infant's death. Their professional reaction was to
explain what did happen and to exert greater professional control over
future birthing situations. First, obstetrical procedures and practices
were reviewed, not just those practiced in the case in question but for
all the births in the practice. Decisions were made to increase use of
medical technologies and interventions. More extensive use of the
fetal heart monitor was initially adopted by the practitioners. Greater
caution, even a hypersensitivity to slight meconium staining (evident
during the birth of the infant who died), became the practice norm.
The standard technology in the women's obstetrical practice had been
use of an external monitoring device, the doptone. The decision to increase use of the fetal monitor was remarkable given the highly elaborated philosophy of low-intervention childbirth for which the practice
was noted. Patients sought care from this physician and her midwife
colleagues *because* of this philosophy and the low-intervention practice
it supported.

Second, the physician and midwives turned to professional colleagues, to the pathologist and to the obstetricians and other midwives
to comment on the case. These consultations were at first informal,
but were followed by a formal case review, when several similar cases
that had been experienced by the obstetricians and midwives in their
practice were reviewed along with this case. All obstetrical cases from
the two practices in which there was evidence of meconium staining
were reviewed and procedures analyzed. The pathologist's report on
the infant's death formally absolved the women of incompetence and
confirmed them in their judgment; it proved to be professionally and
emotionally supportive.

The physician's third professional response was less typical and required unusual personal effort. Several months after the infant's death,
she arranged to attend a university medical center where she spent
several weeks as a trainee with obstetrical specialists. She exposed

herself to the high-risk, high-intervention, high-technology obstetrics that she had earlier abhorred. Ironically, the physician's return to high-risk hospital obstetrics confirmed for her that her philosophy and practice of low-intervention obstetrics was preferable and that her judgment was not impaired.

These three professional modes of coping were highly instrumental actions, oriented to reestablishing a sense of competence and mastery, of control over obstetrical work. They were coupled with much self-reflection and eventually attempts to integrate what had happened into professional as well as personal experience. Yet birthing was a less joyful practice for some time, and the physician relinquished much of the work of delivering babies to her midwifery colleagues. It was only after the mother of the dead infant had a successful birth and healthy child (approximately one year after the first baby's death) that the practice of home births regained most of its equilibrium and emotional satisfaction for several of the practitioners involved. Low-intervention and low-technology obstetrics could be practiced once again without fearing loss of control.

Female and Male; Us and Them

Differences and discrepancies in modes of knowledge, in considerations of what is relevant information and appropriate obstetrical practice, led to a public and professional distinction between "the guys" and "the women," between "us" and "them." This distinction was frequently drawn in public by members of the communities served by these providers as well as within the professional medical community. Patients and medical staff would constantly compare the two groups of obstetrical providers. Articulating this distinction in terms of gender also occurred within both practices, somewhat ironically given that "the guys'" practice included women, the certified nurse-midwives. These women performed the majority of normal deliveries for the obstetricians' practice in the community hospital's family-centered birthing unit; they also assisted the "women" physicians on occasion at home births. The mixing of the two practices, through the work of the midwives and through consultancies the obstetricians performed for the family-practice physicians and independent midwives, led both the men and the women to comment frequently on the practice style and competence of each other. It was not surprising that gender imagery emerged in critical rhetoric and language.

One female practitioner, in discussing these distinctions, identified the "differences between 'us' and 'them'" as rooted in contrasting approaches to obstetrical knowledge. Recalling the case of a woman who had arrested labor for seven hours, she remarked that the obstetricians considered it poor judgment to allow labor to continue without intervention for such long a period. In her view, long labor with good results, "good babies and good bonding . . . are the basis of our consideration." And women who have overcome arrested labor have

feelings about themselves and their ability to relate to their child that has qualitative rewards that I don't think they [the obstetricians] would measure in quite the terms we do. So there are people we have left at home, when somebody would have said objectively that they can't do it, that pit [oxytocin] and forceps are needed. In medical records, it looks ridiculous—seven hours with no progress.

What the male obstetricians can know and what they can't know also constitutes this imaging of "the other."

They don't have the same feeling for it, or as a community of women have for other women. Sure there are areas where they know a lot more than we do. And there are areas where you cannot explain [what is known]. It is as if you are talking a different language. You can't explain it because it is as if there is no *data* to support it. It's very qualitative. We haven't proven that the relationship between a mother and her child is significantly better because that mother found it in her [to overcome an arrested labor] versus another mother who had a forceps delivery and a nice baby. There is no *proof* that bonding is better. It is an entirely *gut* instinctive knowing. And that knowing can only be shared with people who have some place for that understanding through their own experience. A little more of that intuitive experience.

The women did not entirely dismiss the skills of their male colleagues. *Surgical* results were often admired, especially for infertility workups. One woman physician talked about the kind of energy her male colleague invested in his infertility patients.

Now you take his work with his infertility patients—he gives a lot, he gives an arm and a leg. He interrupts vacations, he does things whenever they need to be done, he doesn't give a damn when that is—amazing. He puts his heart and soul into it and he gets incredible results. Amazing.

Similarly, what the women can and cannot know and *do* became part of the critical rhetoric of members of the medical staff. One male physician remarked on the limits that the medical staff's "rules and regulations" set on the women's obstetrical practice by noting that only obstetricians had the right to attend breech and twin births. He felt the women often let patients wait too long before calling the obstetricians but that the interaction between the two groups had as much to do with gender as with specialty.

For whatever their reasons, they do things differently; that probably interferes with communication. . . . They do a lot of things that . . . you know, they're not as well trained as the obstetricians . . . so they do a lot of things, you know, differently. . . . Anyhow, obstetricians only see the problems because if everything else goes fine, they don't get called. . . . [When patients discover they cannot have a home birth and have been allowed to go perhaps too long by the women, the obstetricians] have to be the bad guys. . . . Maybe they have to have a Caesarean or some kind of difficult forceps or something like that—"Well here these guys have to do this uncomfortable stuff." It puts the obstetricians in a difficult situation.

Some women practitioners sought to broaden their privileges and contested the limits the obstetricians sought to impose. Twin births became particularly problematic when one of the women practitioners became pregnant with twins. The obstetricians initially denied her the right to choose who would attend her—she wanted the women from her own practice to provide care rather than one of the obstetricians. Yet the "rules and regulations" governing the medical community prescribed the presence of an obstetrician-surgeon. Women's choice, in providing and consuming obstetrical care, appeared fragile to many women given the presence of specialists in this medical community. Yet the twins were delivered by the woman's partners, while the obstetrician remained unobtrusively out of sight.

The female/male, us/them dichotomy carried a common American cultural refrain that is rich in gender imagery. In the public realm, and at times in the professional medical domain, the women physicians and midwives were identified with having intuitive, qualitative, and experiential knowledge, and the men were considered masters of technological and specialist expertise. Women were skilled in relational matters, men in intervention, doing, and action. Yet the women physicians and midwives, who claimed that their obstetrical knowledge and expertise made them at least as competent as their male colleagues, found these culturally dense gender associations about knowledge, practice, and competence often problematic, conveyers of intensely distressful personal and professional meanings.

Gender Imagery and Competence

Among the three repertoires of discourse on competence I encountered in field research in Coast Community (and elsewhere), the reflective mode compelled me to think through my interpretations about what competence means to physicians (and other clinicians), how these meanings are influenced by our broader cultural contests, and how they affect the work of doctoring. I initially worked out many of the nuances of the personal meanings of competence in a series of intense biweekly conversations with a woman physician who was particularly attuned to gender issues in American culture, in her own thinking, and in that of her medical colleagues. She spoke about many of the professional and personal meanings gender imagery conveys in the contemporary practice of American medicine. Her reflections on competence and gender, while more typical of the generation of women physicians trained in the early 1970s, are remarkable illustrations of how gender imagery becomes deeply entwined in competence discourses in medicine. I carried the insights gained from these conversations to discussions with other physicians and clinicians (and in new research with medical students) and found they resonated regardless of age or gender. They also inform the history of obstetrical/medical politics in Coast Community.

Her reflections are presented largely in her own words (in quotations) and are drawn from the first two years of our ongoing conversation (which continued in a less intense and regular fashion for seven years) on the meaning of competence to physicians. I begin with our earliest conversations when I first opened the discussion on competence, and where she explains how professional competence became wed to and interpreted through personal experiences and values, and proceed to later conversations at the time she became a chief of staff.

Competence is very important to me. I have always half intended to go back and do another residency. What I really wanted to do when I was an intern, the only residency that I looked at and went "oh yum," was a surgery residency. I had two small children. . . . I knew there was just no way, so I did a much shorter residency in family practice. About two years ago, and intermittently since then, I have had attacks of [wanting to do] surgery residencies. I realized from [mulling over] this issue of competence that one of the appeals a surgery residency has for me is that I still have this myth that . . . a good surgeon . . . is the epitome of competence.

The image of a good surgeon, for this woman and for most Americans, is also very *male*.[1] As she went on to analyze why she had these flashes of wishing she could do a surgical residency (recall that obstetrics/gynecology is a surgical as well as medical specialty and, some would argue, a primary-care specialty), she told me:

I am still being run by, without realizing it, my old myth of what competence is. And it's true that many things I used to be really good at have fallen away because I have chosen to go in other directions. And I feel the loss quite keenly. I used to be really good at operating, and now having done less and less over the years, I've gotten more and more incompetent. . . .

    It's just so intimately connected with my strong feelings about competence and my myths about what competence is. . . . I realize that . . . for me as an individual, [I have] newer values of competence. The best thing about a good surgeon is not doing; but the next best thing is doing. I think my old myth around competence was doing. It was . . . something you could see. It was big and dramatic . . . also *very* male. All the things I valued before . . . that is how I *was* before. My style was very out there, very concrete, very doing, very dramatic. Not in the sense that I was dramatic, but that the activity I was engaged in was dramatic.

Placing "doing," "male" images next to the "newer" female images of how to be a physician implied maturity but also losses as well as gains.

I've been working on bringing out other parts of me for a long time. . . . What I've been engaged in by choice, for very conscious reasons, are other things . . . quieter . . . more intuitive . . . not as dramatic . . . much more inward, and I think, female. Much more nurturing. But now, I am beginning to think that the real drive, that resurgence, that strong drive, stronger than ever to do a surgery residency, is at least in part [a reaction to] that polarity. . . . It is a loss of part of myself, a loss of part of myself, my skills, my competence, a valuable part in me. . . . It's so interesting to view this desired activity of mine through the peephole of the issue of competence. It was a whole new light . . . [that helped me feel] less grief and more understanding. Less grief at the loss, more wisdom, more understanding . . . more acceptance.

These reflections brought into focus intensely personal as well as professional issues that were highly gender laden. Like many other women physicians who had children during internship and residency, this physician had not pursued a surgical specialty, although her husband became a surgeon. The course of her professional development therefore deviated from her model of the idealized physician, "the good surgeon." The contrast between what she now valued in herself, professionally and personally, and her "myth" of what epitomizes physician competence, paralleled major changes in her professional and personal life. She moved from an intense and exhausting primary-care practice in the city to a more low-keyed, somewhat alternative practice in a rural area. Her newer emphasis on nurturing led her to choose to act as a catalyst for patients "to bring themselves to wellness." Because of the nature of her new practice, she was able to eschew what she viewed as excessive biotechnology and aggressive medical interventions. This approach was particularly successful in the obstetrical practice she developed with other women. And yet, the gendered "myth" of what epitomizes professional competence and her early images of the ideal physician continued to be extraordinarily powerful as she assessed her personal and professional self and sought to understand her conflicting professional drives. When a newborn's death led her to question her professional performance most seriously, she sought to reassume selected characteristics of her "myth" of what epitomized competence in medicine.

The personal meanings of competence to physicians may have deep roots in childhood experiences and relationships. This same physician, in reflecting on why competence was a "life issue for me," recollected her childhood associations.

Competence was extraordinarily important to my father. He was an engineer, and he was very good at it. My mother was in some respects incompetent. I was always revolted by her incompetence. . . . As long as I can remember, it has been important to me to do things well. . . . It's a real compulsion. I would like to see it become just a part of me and not be so compelling. I'm sure competence was one of the big issues in my own family as a child. . . . I think my father, overtly in his words, validated my competence. My mother validated my competence by her incompetence. She probably validated my father's competence by her incompetence. And she left me with a real rage about incompetent women. A disgust that is male, that is absolutely male. Maybe a travesty of the male, but absolutely male.

Perhaps because the physician associated competence and maleness, her relationships with her male colleagues in obstetrics were particularly complex. But like many other family-practice physicians, she constantly compared her skills and doctoring to the skills and doctoring of specialists in her community.

I think [that] for a long time, I tried to increase my competence, or my vision of myself as competent, or other people's visions of me as competent, at the expense of other physicians' competence. I think that's what a lot of doctors do. It is like there is only so much competence in this world. If I have more, they have less. If they have more, I have less. I think I am just getting to where I don't have to influence people's view of me as competent or my own view of myself as competent, by taking away from somebody else's competence. The mythical part . . . has been my tremendous need to be competent. The reality part is that I am more competent . . . because I am smarter, I care more, I pay more attention. But I am getting to the point, thank God—finally—where I am willing to be competent and there is no necessary comparison. And I am even beginning to speak . . . to someone else's competence. . . . I've eased up on men—other professionals. I think I had a need to put all that out there on someone. And what better than on my *male* colleagues who are *specialists*! If I were a specialist, too, I am sure I would have less need. But I am beginning to appreciate them much more. I still disagree with them a lot. I think there is stuff they miss, but I am not interested in fighting about it. And they are more accepting; . . . they are just not as critical of me.

Elected chief of the medical staff at the community hospital, some years after the baby's death, the physician achieved her position with the support and votes of her male colleagues, including the obstetricians and other surgical specialists.

GENDER AND SPECIALTY

I know sooner or later another confrontation with the OBs is going to come, and that there really is not freedom of choice . . . [a] very painful thing to realize. Ultimately, women don't have choices. Only up to a point because they let us have choices. A woman who is on the staff and cannot choose her own birth attendants—that's shocking.

The feminization of obstetrical practice and care in Coast Community took place in the context of a broad cultural rethinking about birthing in America. It also took place in a changing practice climate for medicine as a profession and for obstetrics and gynecology in particular. The coming of the specialists to rural communities meant that a specialty's rules and regulations, controls and surveillance would also be introduced and become the "standard of care" that measured and insured physician competence. This has been true particularly for the practice of obstetrics in most communities in the United States.

During the late 1970s and early 1980s, many women who were health professionals reinterpreted their own personal and professional experiences with birthing. The reflective knowledge gained through this reinterpretation was often channeled into passionate reform, into both intraprofessional and public discourse and actions to alter the meaning of the birthing experience. The possibilities that personal experiences could be reinterpreted and linked to action to reform obstetrical care must be considered as part of the context of the prevailing women's health and birthing movements of the era. This broader cultural rethinking allowed for the realization of opportunities for home births and alternative birth experiences. The tolerance within the new specialty of family medicine for performing home births, the state's response to the popular demand for alternative births through the introduction of certified training programs and licensure in midwifery (despite resistance from organized medicine), and the acceptance, if at times grudging, by obstetrical specialists of alternative forms and locations of births (often with agreements to provide hospital consultations if necessary), provided the prerequisites for these changes in the birthing experience and in birth choices. Clearly the individual practitioners who created alternative choices in birthing profited from these broader cultural movements and social responses even as they initiated, formulated, and contributed to them. Yet choice is but "allowed," as the physician quoted above noted. The medical profession, the state, and individual practitioners and patients create constraints to practice and reform. In American society, such constraints are often attributed to specialty interests and gendered behavior. When the climate of practice is altered, when crises provoked by changes in the political economy of medicine erupt, achievements liberalizing practice are subject to reconsideration and gains may be quickly lost. In 1985, a malpractice crisis threatened obstetrical care on the coast and shook the medical community to its very core.

CHAPTER FOUR

A Crisis of Competence

*And when they got sued, they were just completely
disrupted. They thrashed around and spun it off on
everyone else.*

—A family practice physician, female

*We went from being the good guys and really doing
something for the community, . . . getting all the positive
feedback one gets from delivering babies, to sort of being
the bad guys. But in a way we were, because we started
discussing how we were going to deal with the other
practitioners.*

—An obstetrician, male

In late 1985, a malpractice suit was brought against the
obstetricians who practiced in Coast Community. The doctors felt
stunned, professionally threatened, and financially vulnerable. The alternative and rural ethos of the region had led many physicians to go
without malpractice insurance when they first entered practice there.
Before the suit, the obstetricians, who had no malpractice insurance at
the time, formed contractual agreements with individual patients; each
patient who entered their care acknowledged acceptance of the lack of
malpractice insurance and its implications. The midwives who practiced
with the obstetricians had malpractice coverage, but it was limited, and
one of the family physicians who practiced obstetrics had malpractice
insurance. At the time of the suit, her premiums cost one-fifth of what

the obstetricians would eventually have to pay. An assumption of trust and good will between most physicians and their patients led many young physicians "to go bare." Thus, the malpractice suit came as a great surprise.

The suit was brought by a woman who lost her infant to preterm hemorrhaging and premature birth despite medical evacuation to a metropolitan teaching hospital. Among the medical community and among most of the interested public, the suit was considered to be a spoiler and unfounded. However, the malpractice suit precipitated an ominous series of events that led to a deeply troubling "crisis of competence." As negotiations wound through the legal system over the course of eighteen months, the region's obstetrical providers were thrown into turmoil.

The uniqueness of this local crisis of competence was in part shaped by the correlation of gender with specialty—of maleness with obstetrical specialists, and of femaleness with the family practice physicians and midwives, even though midwives were associated with both specialties. Because gender and specialty overlapped, debates over what constituted quality obstetrical care and over the appropriate hierarchy of expertise, responsibility, and control were heightened and colored by gender imagery. In the previous chapter I discussed how these gender differences were interpreted in terms of kinds of knowledge brought to practice, and through the ideology and philosophy of birthing. Philosophies of birthing were linked to issues of hierarchy and control because the women practiced home births out of the immediate purview and domain of the specialists, thus defying easy control and monitoring by the obstetricians. The alternative practices of the women providers were considered by some physicians to be potentially "risky" for the obstetricians, their specialist consultants.

Suddenly, when the obstetricians were sued, their concerns about "risk" and "competence" transformed what had been a somewhat uneasy but generally collegial consultant relationship with the women practitioners. The malpractice suit cast that relationship into a crisis that reflected larger national developments in obstetrics and in the medical profession. Soaring costs for liability insurance, increasingly divisive conflicts between family medicine and obstetrics, changing demographics and density of physicians, and problems of access to and financing of obstetrical care—all were making the practice of obstetrics exceedingly difficult throughout the country. Therefore even though the local crisis was a "diagnostic and documentary event" revealing the ideological and economic cleavages and the cultural conflicts among the *local* community of physicians and patients, it also exemplified the reasons why there was a national crisis in obstetrical care[1] (see chapter 5).

The Malpractice Crisis

Initially, the obstetricians reacted to the malpractice claim by frantically seeking support from the state, the community, the hospital, and their medical colleagues, to pay for malpractice insurance. They threatened *there would be no obstetrics on the coast* if a satisfactory solution to the problem could not be found. They defined the malpractice problem as one affecting not only themselves but all providers of obstetrical care, the hospital and medical staff, and the women who sought to give birth in the community. Someone would have to reimburse them for their *professional risk taking,* for simply *practicing obstetrics,* and for providing consultative backup for the family physicians and midwives. Most of their medical colleagues responded negatively to the obstetricians' attempts to get the Coast hospital to pay for their malpractice insurance, either on a per-patient basis or as "employees" of the district hospital. As the community of physicians had grown through the decade to over thirty-five doctors, malpractice insurance had increasingly become the norm for the medical staff at Coast hospital. And it was expected that one day the obstetricians would also have to pay their dues. As one doctor commented, "the hospital doesn't pay my malpractice insurance; why should it pay theirs!"

Yet early in the crisis, the obstetricians earned some sympathy and support from their colleagues, for in spite of the simmering "turf" battles between the male specialists and female family physicians and midwives, the obstetricians *had* created a revolution in birthing for the region. In addition, the exchanges, referrals, and consultations between specialists and generalists continued to function quite reasonably into mid-decade, there was enough business for all, and the midwives continued to mediate between the competing practices and specialties of the female and male physicians, thus smoothing these professional relationships.

A woman physician, reflecting on the way the obstetricians first responded to the suit, sympathized with their distress: they "were just completely disrupted. They thrashed around and spun it off on every-one else." But she speculated on how they should have expressed their feelings. Instead of anger and attack, she felt they could have more effectively gained support from their colleagues and the community through expressing their hurt.

If I could have legislated the way I thought it should have been, they would have gone "Ooow—this hurts! This is *horrible*! We have given good service to this community and have set up a *model* program here. We've given of our-selves to such an extent, that the women . . . who have had babies in this community have *no idea* what it is like elsewhere! I think we should send them to [the city]." (Late fall, year one of the crisis)

The situation soon deteriorated further, however, and by the fall the women physicians dissolved their partnership. One continued in partnership with the midwife with whom she had worked for most of her professional career on the coast; they returned to maintaining a small and select practice, known to some as a "Cadillac practice." The second family practice physician recruited a certified nurse-midwife from the city, and she expanded her obstetrical practice considerably. Competition of significant economic consequence arose shortly after the malpractice suit. A long-time member of the medical community recalled the turmoil this new economically significant competition was soon to bring about, given the embattled state of the obstetricians.

When she came [the new midwife], I knew the shit was going to hit the fan! There were too many practitioners here for the number of people. The specter of competition reared its ugly head. And there are some other things that reared their ugly head! The doctors had gone without malpractice insurance for years and years. And then they were sued. And they realized how vulner-able they were. When they first came here, they did not have very much. And now they *do*. And they were vulnerable to losing it. And that meant getting malpractice insurance, which costs a small fortune. (Summer, second year of the crisis)

As the obstetricians began to strike out at other providers in response to the suit, one of the family physicians for whom the OBs had will-ingly provided backup recalled how the traditional consultancy rela-tionship began to change.

They . . . started doing all that stuff to us, . . . essentially saying, "We can't back you up, because we are having enough trouble of our own." And just prior to that [the woman family physician] had had many more patients and many more complications. (Summer, year two of the crisis)

The crisis of competence was beginning to take shape; it was on the verge of unfolding in all its destructiveness.

STRATEGIES AND CONSEQUENCES

The obstetricians, with the assistance of their midwives, soon began aggressively pursuing a variety of strategies to compensate for the cost of malpractice premiums. Assistance and intervention was sought from state legislators and health committees, and state aid and grant possibilities were explored. A number of funding schemes were proposed to the district hospital board, including one in which the hospital would employ the obstetricians to conduct deliveries just as it employed other local physicians, on an hourly basis, to cover the emergency room. This scheme and others were debated in public meetings of the hospital board; the rooms were often packed with hospital and medical staff and the public, including many pregnant women and health activists, and tempers were hot. Through these public debates, the obstetricians continued to hold out the threat to withdraw from obstetrical practice and discontinue obstetrical backup for the midwives and family physicians if the hospital and community did not help them resolve their difficulties.

The malpractice crisis thus became a very public drama. Professional conflicts, previously enacted exclusively within the bounds of professional discourse, were acted out and debated in public forums and in the region's press. In a very real sense, through their aggressive stance and threat to withhold their expertise and skills, the obstetricians lost the sympathy of a community they had served long and well. For some members of the community, their moral authority was seriously compromised. One obstetrician reflected on how he felt during the crisis:

The one thing that hit me, that I didn't like, was that we went from being the good guys and really doing something for the community, . . . getting all the positive feedback one gets from delivering babies, to sort of being the bad guys. But in a way we were, because we started discussing how we were going to deal with the other practitioners. . . . I didn't feel the need, that we needed to have a *lot* of support from all the people, at the same time that we were getting sued, but somehow that lack of feeling from the community did hurt a little bit. (Summer, year two of the crisis)

Although the obstetricians hoped to receive sympathy and political support by making their case public, they learned the dangers of taking discussions traditionally confined to professional contexts into the public arena.

When the hospital board found it extremely difficult—legally, administratively, and financially—to accept any of the proposed malpractice financing schemes, the obstetricians escalated their threat. They took a public and political stance and declared they would not offer obstetrical services to the community: there would be no consultative backup to other providers; Medi-Cal patients were no longer welcomed in their practice; their practice would be limited to gynecology. The obstetricians created a situation in which *there would be no authorized obstetrics on the coast.* The physicians intended to use this stance to pressure the state and the hospital to redress the local malpractice crisis and to assist them with their financial burden. But as they waited for the state to respond to grant applications developed by their midwives, which would eventually provide special coverage for Medi-Cal patients, their relationship with the other obstetrical providers and with the community deteriorated precipitously.

One member of the medical community recounted the situation at this point:

When they stopped practicing OB, and they did stop taking OB patients for a month, their gynecology dropped off just like that! Their book was just empty, they were walking around twiddling their thumbs. They thought, well they could just continue gynecology and somehow survive that way. It was obvious that the two go hand in hand. There is a lot of spin-off GYN that you get from your obstetrical practice. I think there was manipulation there too. But I also think they seriously wanted to see—what's going to happen if we do this. And I think they were stunned by the response.

After several months, the doctors realized they could not survive without practicing obstetrics and offering the option for low-intervention/low-risk obstetrics practiced by their midwives. *Thus, in midstruggle, they purchased private malpractice insurance.*

Although they took the step of purchasing insurance, for seven months the obstetricians continued to refuse to accept Medi-Cal patients in their practice as they sought to lobby the state into action. The state at the time paid only $480 per patient for prenatal care and hospital delivery; the obstetricians had calculated that their costs for private malpractice insurance alone averaged $300 per patient. These were not unreasonable calculations. Thus, the doctors hoped that the other obstetrical providers would support them in their political efforts. But the reaction of some community members, including pregnant women who were on Medi-Cal, was vociferous and negative. The obstetricians were accused of being against the poor women of the coast! There was irony in the accusation, given that prior to the suit the obstetricians and their midwives willingly took care of Medi-Cal patients, who made up approximately one-third of their practice, and their negotiations with the state were intended to gain special coverage for Medi-Cal patients that would include additional nutritional programs as part of prenatal care.

As the men took their case to the state and to the public, one of the women family physicians continued to offer obstetrical care and home births to Medi-Cal patients, some of whom had been turned away from the obstetricians' practice, ostensibly referred to the county-staffed hospital some two hours distant. The obstetricians became incensed at this physician, whom they perceived as breaking ranks with the rest of the obstetrical providers on the coast, especially when they began to assess the decline in their overall patient population and the extraordinary increase in her obstetrical cases. In the year prior to the malpractice suit, she had had five to six deliveries per month; after the suit, when a new midwife joined her, deliveries increased to ten to twelve per month.

Competition now had far more serious consequences given the obstetricians' need to pay malpractice premiums. The doctors had hoped soon to recoup a full complement of patients, and as previously, to fill their practice and that of their midwives. They found that the newly formed practice of their female colleague and the arrival of a new midwife partner eroded that possibility. A colleague of the obstetricians and the family practice physician recounted the men's reaction.

The docs wanted everybody to pull together to try to get subsidization for the Medi-Cal patients, for the malpractice insurance. [The woman family physician] took—in some people's view—an unfair opportunity to take on the patients the doctors were refusing to see. And they *were* doing that—that was definitely manipulative—trying to manipulate the state into giving them additional monies for those Medi-Cal patients. And see, what [she] did [by taking those patients] was completely undermining what [the obstetricians] were doing. . . . It was a chance to increase her practice and serve as a shining light. And of course the guys were pissed purple.

LEGALIZING ANGER

The obstetricians acted upon their anger. They informed all obstetrical providers that they would not give obstetrical consultation and backup unless their colleagues paid them $300 per patient. Ostensibly, the obstetricians argued, they placed themselves at "risk" when they cared for the women's patients and even when they simply were available for these patients. In particular, they argued, the economically "at-risk" and perhaps "medically high-risk" Medi-Cal patients of their chief competitor put them at "professional risk." They wanted to be compensated for the costs of protection against that risk. Without consultant backup, the obstetrical privileges of the family physicians and midwives were threatened. This action created a furor in the broader medical community. It was considered undoctorly, unprofessional, illegal, and an infringement on the right to practice. One of the women providers threatened to bring a lawsuit against the obstetricians for unlawful restriction of practice in response to the obstetricians' legal maneuvers to extract payment and a contract and their refusal to provide consultation backup.

Negotiations conducted through the medical staff and others brought an interim resolution; the obstetricians would be paid $300 per patient; each patient would be seen once or twice, and the fee would be credited to any necessary care delivered in the hospital. The agreement barely settled the turmoil and continued to be viewed as an irritant, only marginally legal, by many in the medical community, including, of course, the women providers of obstetrical care. The legal display of anger played out over months, and it further complicated the practice of obstetrics on the coast.

A Crisis of Competence and the Language of Risk

The obstetricians found themselves on the defensive in their professional and legal relationship with the other physicians and midwives. They sought to correct this by appealing to what they perceived as being medically justified and a higher moral ground. They went to the public to explain why they wished to be paid *per patient* to provide specialty consultation. And in doing so, they questioned the competence of the nonspecialists. This public appeal proved to have grave consequences for all concerned. It confounded medical competence, competition, and the meaning of risk in a highly volatile public and political debate. At the peak of the crisis, when the obstetricians were still not taking Medi-Cal patients and when they were in the middle of quite acrimonious contract negotiations with the women, one partner wrote an open letter to a local community newspaper. It utilized the language of risk, the very choice of which was infused with implications of the specialist's power and right to judge and control the practice of the generalist. I have italicized the language of risk as used in this letter and as reproduced by other medical professionals in interviews I conducted during the height of the crisis.

An open letter from a specialist in obstetrics/gynecology:

One practitioner in the community, in my opinion, has compromised patient safety by caring for *high-risk patients*. . . . When recent problems have developed in patients I felt were *high-risk*, I felt that I, in good conscience and closed mouth, could no longer continue with the "status quo." Physicians have been ordered to "police themselves"; however, recently when I decided that I could *no longer legitimize practices which I felt contained lapses of good medical judgment*, and withdrew my being available for "backup" to this practitioner, I was threatened with a *lawsuit and restraining order*. (Spring, year one of the crisis)

What lay behind this extraordinary breach of professional boundaries and traditional ethics? Spilling a professional conflict into the public domain was clearly a "risky" activity in itself. The community's medical professionals—physicians, midwives, nurses—attempted to puzzle out what motivated the obstetricians' politically risky behavior. Again, the language and rhetoric of "competence" and "risk" is symbolically central to the conflict and emerged in discussions and public comments by members of the medical community. Midwives and physicians, supporters of the practitioner who became the focus of the obstetricians' anger, supporters of the obstetricians, and those who found themselves arbiters for both, framed their analyses in similar ways. A midwife:

Well, all of a sudden she was a whole lot busier, and I think that was difficult for her to deal with, covering all the bases became real difficult. And when she became the focus of their anger and frustration, they began attacking her. And everyone would have said—is there any truth to these [accusations of incompetence]?
[Question: Has she ever had any infant deaths? Bad babies?]
Not that I know of.

A physician negotiator:

The feeling of the OB guys was that [V.] was taking on more difficult patients than she could—that she really should not be managing *high-risk* obstetrics.

[Question: Any infant deaths? Bad outcomes?]
Not evidently.

A family physician:

She had many more patients and many more complications. . . . You can't take *high-risk people* and expect to come out with a *no-risk situation*.
[Question: Any dead babies?]
Uh, un. No-o-o-o.
[Question: What leads one into these high-risk situations? Such as allowing a high-risk patient to try a home birth?]
This is a problem which [we] get into very often, which is absorbing other people's [patients'] considerations which oughtn't to be properly absorbed by us. . . . I wasn't critical of her, because I've done it so many times—I knew what happened—she got trapped by absorbing the woman's considerations. . . . The worse situation you can be in.

The physician continued:

Now the OBs, and the other doctors who are male, and this is a particularly female failing—*they don't do that ever*. So they have no—they call it poor medical judgment. It is not poor medical judgment—they have no feeling for it because they don't do it and they don't even know when someone's doing it because it is so far from where they sit.

Physicians whose boundaries are permeable to patients' concerns appear more likely to incur professional difficulties as they adjust their practice decisions to patients' wishes. Among many women on the coast, the prevailing ethos held that home births were highly desirable and achievable. The "standards" for the lay community at times differed from those of the specialists. In such situations, the "standards" of obstetrical practice for high-risk patients can be negotiated and influenced by the quality of the doctor-patient relationship. In the context of the crisis of competence, the accusation that the family practitioner privileged patients' considerations over traditional obstetrical decision making was held as evidence of questionable medical judgment.

Lay supporters of the family practitioner responded through the local and regional press and in an angry community meeting. Many had given birth under her care. They were incensed and viewed the obstetricians' behavior as engaging in gender politics. News stories captured the public dimensions of the conflict and associated the attack on the family physician with the less public and virulent critiques of all women obstetrical providers. Anger was articulated in the language of gender opposition. A community news essay:

Rumors have been mounted that certain general practitioners and midwives are incompetent. The alleged incompetents are seeing increased numbers of pregnant patients who feel more comfortable in the hands of women than they do men. (Spring, year one of the crisis)

A regional press story on the crisis:

Many women viewed them [the male obstetricians] as selfish, uncaring symbols of the male medical establishment—in contrast to Dr. [V.] . . . who seemed to embody female generosity and dedication. (Fall, year one of the crisis)

A year after the onslaught and after legal negotiations had brought a modicum of quiet and resolution to the crisis, the besieged practitioner reflected on how she had come to be embroiled in a public battle with the obstetricians. She marshaled a defense, articulating it in the language of competence, mirroring the accusations and language of her competitors and justifying her style of practice in terms of obstetrical competence, judgment, and considerations of *risk*.

They spent a lot of energy to get me on some case. . . . It was very scary, because I do practice somewhat different [medicine], want things done a little bit differently. . . . I had patients . . . who left their practice. When [the obstetricians] were warned [she had threatened legal action over unlawful restriction of practice], there was really no case that they could say . . . there was real mismanagement. . . . It's like apples and oranges. It can be—okay, here in this case you might have written a little longer note, or something relatively minor. *That in no way could be construed, ever, as incompetence. Or poor management, or something like that.*

I never lost a baby, knock on wood, I mean ever. In all the seven years, I've never lost a baby here. . . . Part of it is I am lucky. . . . God is on my side, . . . but I feel like I have done a really good job. *I have this great instinct about knowing who could be a problem and doing things early on, being real aggressive at that time.* . . . There is no greater mortality and morbidity in home births, in fact . . . they are supposed to be safer according to some studies if you choose *low-risk* patients.

The family practitioner's colleagues felt they could legitimately engage in speculating on her competence because she challenged the boundaries of practice defined by the specialists. Her apparent willingness to accept high-risk patients for home births, including patients rejected by the "Cadillac" practice of the other women providers, potentially placed "at malpractice risk" the obstetrical consultants who were required to provide backup for these patients. Although none of the patients referred by any of the women practitioners to the obstetricians for emergency surgical procedures, for Caesarean or breech deliveries, had ever entertained or brought malpractice suits against the specialists, the obstetricians were acutely sensitive to potential risk. In their view, the family practitioner's assumption of care for a patient whom *they* would define as "high risk" created a risky situation with potential bad outcomes. And they feared the possibility of malpractice suits as attending consultants.

The language of risk also provided a medically authorized way to critique the physician's judgment, in terms of apparent *practice* and potential consequences rather than an evaluation of *outcome*. Perhaps most clearly, it became a medically moralized language and rhetoric through which "the specter of competition could rear its ugly head" and be professionally masked.

Specialty and Gender Confounded

Boundaries between medicine practiced, authorized, and regulated by specialists and that practiced by nonspecialists are frequently defined and debated in the language of "risk." Obstetrics calls upon generalists, family medicine physicians, and midwives to limit practice to low-risk patients and low-intervention, low-technology birthing. All three disciplines—obstetrics, family medicine, and midwifery—through their national and academic societies and colleges—dispute and contest the boundaries that circumscribe their domains of practice. The language of risk is central to these professional debates. (Family medicine, as a discipline, has challenged the obstetrical specialists' definition of a high-risk patient. See chapter 5.) Michael Klein, a family medicine professor who writes extensively about obstetrics for family medicine, commented that for obstetricians to be satisfied, a low-risk woman must be "bionic"; family physicians "will soon need a consult to perform vaginal births." [Seminar, Department of Social Medicine, Harvard Medical School, November 1990] Thus, it was not surprising that in the local "crisis of competence," highly diverse meanings of "risk" from medical *and* popular culture became core idioms in the providers' struggle to define their own "authorized" practice. Because "risk" defined as "risky practices" and "risky birthing contexts" came to be associated with women providers who were not specialists, the obstetricians' efforts to define what constituted high- and low-risk obstetrics and who had the authority to attend at high-risk births became confounded with the politics of gender.[2]

In this crisis of competence, the obstetricians legitimated their efforts to control and curtail the practice of their nonspecialist competitors by invoking recent changes in the guidelines and standards published by the American College of Obstetrics and Gynecology (ACOG).
Their legitimacy to enact these changes was conveyed through the
power of organized specialty and academic medicine. Rules and regulations delineating hospital obstetrical privileges and procedures were
revised and accepted without serious debate by the local medical staff
and hospital administration. This process was viewed with dismay by
the female family physician. She recalled that the American Academy
of Family Practice (AAFP) disputes many ACOG regulations that were
instituted with the change. The AAFP-ACOG disagreements have generated intense debate over practice boundaries and meanings of "risk"
within the centers of medical education and residency training as well
as among local medical communities.[3]

In Coast Community, the struggle between the specialists and the
family practitioners took another hostile turn when local rules and
regulations governing obstetrical privileges at the district hospital were
reformulated. The obstetricians sought to reassert control over their
threatened practice domain by continuing the discourse on competence and risk. One midwife remarked about the near inviolability of
the obstetrical hierarchy, even after the moral stance of the specialists
was called into question by the public and by supporters of the woman
family physician.

It's the hierarchy thing. The obstetrician is the top dog and he automatically
becomes head of OB and supervises everybody else.
    [Question: And writes the rules?]
    Right, exactly. They have a lot of power here because they have a total
monopoly [in the district]. They are all in one practice; they're *the only
practice.*

One of the obstetricians, in reflecting on his response to the crisis and
that of his specialist colleagues recalled:

Our rules and regulations have been really tightened up . . . and certain procedures, like pitocin. The obstetrician on call *has to be notified* it is going to
happen. It can't just happen, . . . I came in for fetal distress while pitocin was
running. Especially in view of the fact that you might have an immediate
problem, that the OB may have to do a Caesarean section. . . . It is not just
our rules—these are the rules that come from the American College of Obstetrics and Gynecology "Standards of Practice." . . . It says . . . if an induction is
to be started, somebody who has the ability to do an operative delivery should

be available. Now you could say we are using that for our own benefit. The American Academy of Family Practice is debating that whole thing.

The very practices and technologies of contemporary obstetrics that monitor and survey mother and infant also monitor and control the practitioner (Arney 1982:99–154). When "monitoring practices" are generated and defined by one's own specialty, they legitimate and authorize one's position within the local medical hierarchy. Through this authorization specialists acquire the power and mechanisms to control and regulate not only mothers and the birthing process but other practitioners as well. Such regulation ostensibly serves to improve and standardize medical practices and to assure the quality of care given to patients. These are worthy, important goals. Yet, in some cases, regulation can appear primarily to sharpen interspecialty rivalry or to serve the interests of one specialty over against those of another. Monitoring techniques and regulations (use of the fetal monitor is but one among many; record keeping is among the most critical) for some practitioners, especially the nonspecialist, are anathema. Ideologically these monitoring procedures may be negatively characterized as "interfering" in the natural process of birthing; but perhaps they become most threatening to physicians when they are perceived as vehicles of interference with and external control of one's own medical practices. When physicians feel that they are practicing competent, high-quality medicine, such surveillance can be experienced as a hostile interference from the dominant specialty.

One of the female family physicians commented on the changes in the rules and regulations governing obstetrical practice in the local district hospital, changes that were instituted after the malpractice suit was brought and the crisis of competence began to unfold. She perceived these changes as unwarranted and as personally and politically motivated—the men's response to the competitive atmosphere that had, for the moment, poisoned the provider community.

They did change the rules and regulations so *I* would have to consult them on things I did not have to consult on before. And they said the reason was that JCAH[4] came down with some new guidelines, but they are only guidelines, you see. To have me consult every time I use pitocin, and it turns out one-third of all hospital patients get pitocin. . . . they would have the option of coming in, seeing the patient and deciding if I was fit to manage that patient. *Now that's one-third of my hospital patients,* that they decided—[they] could take over management.

[Question: What do you think is going on? Is this a control issue, not just money?]

That's right. It is at all different levels, and a lot of it is control. And a lot of it comes from fear of all kinds. I don't know why other people have to control other people. My dealings with them . . . [show] how they act, how they are condescending. I went to a perinatal conference . . . two months ago . . . and I probably know as much theoretical OB in many areas as they do.

The interspecialty rivalry that led to questions about practitioners' professional competence and care for patients was deeply distressing to both male and female physicians. The desire to perform well, to demonstrate one's competence, knowledge, and skill, and to be considered a caring physician are part of medicine's professional and ideal persona, of what it means to be a doctor. Clearly for the woman family practitioner, the attacks by the specialists stung her core sense of competence. She exclaimed she *knew* she was an intelligent physician; she argued that she practiced obstetrics "at least as well as the guys," but she felt compelled to attend conferences in perinatal obstetrics to demonstrate that she was as knowledgeable as those who reviewed her practice and controlled her privileges. And in acts of resistance to the specialists' regulations, she challenged their efforts to control her hospital practice by calling for consultations at the last moment, thus often performing difficult deliveries such as breech births independently and with success, before the consulting physician could arrive. These acts of challenge and resistance and attempts at dramatic displays of obstetrical competence were greeted with dismay by the obstetricians and by other medical colleagues.

Male as well as female physicians grew deeply distressed as gender politics colored their struggles. Imagery that had previously distinguished the practices of the men and the women in a tolerable and at times amusing manner gave way to increasingly hostile characterizations following the suit and the unfolding of the crisis. The male specialists, who had indeed been regarded as "white knights" when they first revolutionized birthing on the coast, found that their public images as caring, alternative physicians were sullied and questioned. Although the community of women—their potential patients—might continue to associate maleness and specialty with technical knowledge and skill, maleness had also come to mean aggressiveness, "self-serving interests," and hostile control over female practitioners. Some women feared that the "hostile control" over women practitioners might also extend to women patients, intruding on patient autonomy and restricting women's choices in the orchestration of the birthing process.

This cultural tenor pervaded the community for some time, and the male obstetricians expressed unease at crossing the gender line. One physician related his dismay over changes in the obstetricians' image from "chivalrous knight" to "unwelcome technician." Originally quoted in a regional news story, he repeated the same comment to me in an interview a year later: "When I came here I thought I was on the side of Lancelot; now I find out I am one of the bad guys" (Summer, year two of the crisis). When speaking about his fear of having to provide consultative backup for the women practitioners, he fretted:

Plus, whenever they had a problem, they would hold onto it until the very last minute, and we would get thrown into it. *And people don't really want me to call the shots, all of a sudden; you can't establish credibility in thirty seconds. They don't know you. And, in fact, they have chosen* not *to go see you because you represent organized technical skills that they are not interested in.* (Summer, year two of the crisis)

Issues of gender may have been far more salient in the crisis of competence that occurred on the coast than in medical disputes elsewhere in the country, and recent changes in the demographic profile of obstetricians, with many more women in residency programs, will increasingly shift the association between gender and specialty. In part, the intensity of gender conflicts during the crisis may be attributed to the obstetrical context of the crisis. Disagreements between the male specialists and female generalists over what constituted authorized practice, appropriate medical interventions, and low-risk home births and over how to consider and evaluate patients' wishes and concerns were readily expressed in terms of gender and competence. These debates were by no means limited to the physicians and midwives engaged in the crisis; they were of major interest to the community at large as evidenced by the press attention and the pregnant women who demonstrated at public and hospital meetings. Community gossip focused on the crisis for many months. And *because* the key professional actors in this community were male specialists and female generalists—who served female patients—disputes over power and control of obstetrical practice were quickly expressed in the language of gender opposition. Female nurturance and consideration of patients' needs were contrasted with the standard regulations of the male specialists. Male technical skills and thus instrumental competence were posed against female expressive competence. The resistance of women practitioners to specialty surveillance, definitions of high risk, and delineations of practice boundaries were cast as a struggle for control between the women and the men.

Gendered distinctions wedded to professional performance take on intensely personal meanings that are fundamental not only to the struggle for professional identity and worth but to one's position within the hierarchy of medicine and one's freedom to practice. As the comments of physicians and midwives illustrate, much of the personal anguish of the crisis was intensified because it was articulated in terms of male-female opposition and competing articulations of "symbolic competence."

An Ethnographic Update: Obstetrics in Coast Community

The physicians and midwives felt beleaguered by the crisis of competence as it continued to unfold. Much of the passion and knowledge that each had brought to obstetrical care was lost, in part because of the local crisis and in part because of the difficulties posed by the looming crisis in medical liability. The national malpractice crisis not only intensified economic competition and specialty cleavages among providers of obstetrical care but also led to a cultural crisis within medicine itself. The fundamental cultural ideals of American medicine—the caring dimensions of practice that were beneficial to patients and gave community physicians personal gratification in their work—had been grounded in the assumption of "trust" between patients and physicians and specialty consultants. The ideal of "trust" between physician and patient, characteristically American, can be undermined through situations that create legal adversaries, neither appropriately compensating patients nor efficiently controlling the quality of care. One obstetrician reflected on how the malpractice suit brought about a dramatic change in how he felt about his work:

One [result] is the question of your competency. Once you deal with that, and you say, I know I didn't do anything wrong, *then* you have the whole question of your trust in other people. People come to see you and they trust you. At the same time you trust them. It's a strange feeling—boy I gave this lady a hug the last time I saw her, and now she's suing me. Who do I trust? Who else, who's next?

The obstetrical community arrived at an interim resolution, and the obstetricians agreed to cross the gender line and provide consultations and hospital coverage through contract to each of the family practitioners and midwives. This quasi-legal arrangement continued in force for the next several years. However, the crisis produced serious disaffection among the obstetrical community. One of the women physicians left the community several years after the crisis began to unfold to enter a subspecialty program in a distant city. A second physician radically reduced the size of her practice and within the year discontinued the practice of obstetrics. By the end of the decade she had left the community. One of the male obstetricians temporarily moved to a metropolitan hospital to practice high-technology gynecology and to increase his specialty skills in fertility surgery. Several of the lay midwives who were birth attendants at many home deliveries found other compelling work in education to which they could bring their knowledge and passion. The independent certified nurse-midwives continue to be popular and to practice with medical coverage provided by other physicians and specialty consultations provided by the remaining obstetricians. They continue to offer home births. The certified nurse-midwives who worked with the obstetricians continue to do so, and are much sought after by pregnant women on the coast. By the turn of the decade, hierarchies of specialty and gender were gradually reasserted and reinstitutionalized, at least for the historical moment.

MEANING AND POWER

This ongoing medical event epitomized the local crisis in medical authority, hierarchy, and competence at a time of macro–social change in American medicine, and revealed the multiplicity of voices that exists among communities of practicing physicians. The profession of medicine, which in the simplest version of critical analysis is portrayed as unitary, appears far less so when examined in ethnographic detail. The crisis of competence, as a diagnostic and documentary event, challenges singular views of the medical world and unitary definitions of competence in medical practice. Definitions of competence and risk and the structure of authority to control such definitions are matters of enormous consequence and thus of political struggle. Power, knowledge—and gender—are deeply entwined.

The fragility of American medical communities is illustrated by this particular case, but this case is not atypical of American medicine. Neither is the deep interdependence of the "medical periphery" and the "medical center" of life in local medical communities and in academic medical centers. In the local community described here, as competence talk was mobilized against the family practitioners and midwives, appeals were made to the symbolic core of American medicine. Standards of practice, appropriate procedures, competent management of high-risk patients, rules and regulations—competence language generated from the centers of medical training and from the publications of the boards of medical specialties—came to dominate disputes over authorized practice, collegial and consultative obligations, and structures of specialty power. This symbolic discourse imparted a particular intensity to the crisis. "Competence talk," laden as it was with the symbolic power of the core cultural icons of American medicine, articulated and responded to two contemporary macro–social changes: the national medical malpractice crisis and the transformation of the gender profile of the profession. The implications of these changes for the meaning of obstetrical competence and care are discussed in the next chapter.

CHAPTER FIVE

National Crises in Obstetrical Care

Competence and Risk Reexamined

Local events often presage as well as reflect national movements and trends. The crisis of competence described in the previous chapter, although intensely local, unfolded in parallel with the emerging national crisis in obstetrical practice. During the 1980s, obstetricians throughout the country protested the rising costs of medical liability premiums; physicians went on strike, withdrew from practice, and questioned the unprecedented rise in malpractice claims. Fears circulated as women wondered who would provide obstetrical care. Newspapers were filled with accounts of medicine's protests, and professionals, the public, and state legislatures were baffled at this ominous shift in the environment of medical and obstetrical practice.[1] Efforts by individual physicians, organized medicine, and specialty groups from obstetrics and family practice to stem the malpractice tide led to a redefinition of "risk" and to programs in "risk management." And women throughout the country began to encounter barriers to quality obstetrical care as physicians responded to the early stage of the crisis by limiting "high-risk" obstetrics and care for "high-risk" patients, or by dropping out of obstetrical practice entirely.

Initially, in the years 1982–1985, the crisis appeared primarily to be confined to the specialty of obstetrics. However, as in Coast Community, the tensions created by malpractice claims quickly spilled over to affect obstetrical care offered by family physicians and nurse-midwives.

As these tensions erupted, differences between the specialties of obstetrics and family medicine were articulated in terms of professional competence, and the consultancy relationship suffered under the strain of apparent embattlement. The meaning of competence became an issue around which many conflicts coalesced. What was on the horizon for obstetrical practice as the national malpractice crisis became full-blown by mid-decade?[2]

National Trends

Four major developments in medicine during the 1980s contributed to an intensification of interest in obstetrical competence. There was (1) a generational change in the demographic profile of physicians, in terms of numbers, age, sex, and training; (2) a "malpractice" crisis that threatened obstetrical coverage, particularly in community hospitals and rural settings; (3) a serious review of "standards of practice" and definitions of risk by the American College of Obstetrics and Gynecology and the American Board of Family Practice, in order to strengthen "risk-management" procedures, control liability, and stem the tide of provider attrition; and (4) a continuing debate about ideal modes of birthing, carried on in part by patients and the women's health movement and in part by physicians and midwives concerned with the quality of obstetrical care.

Demographic Profiles: Generational Changes

A generational change of major magnitude occurred in the demographic profile of the medical profession in the United States. The number of physicians almost doubled, from 334,028 in 1970 to 653,062 by 1992. The physician-to-population ratio rose from 161 per 100,000 in 1970 to 255 per 100,000 in 1992 (American Medical Association 1993) and was accompanied by concomitant changes in the age, training, specialty, and gender of physicians. These demographic changes provide one structural key to understanding the national crisis in obstetrical care.

GENERATIONAL DISTINCTIONS: AGE AND TRAINING

The coming of the specialists and residency-trained primary care physicians to rural medical communities coincided with a shift out of general practice and into family medicine. In 1986, approximately 63 percent of physicians who designated themselves as general practitioners were over the age of fifty-five and almost one-third were over the age of sixty-five; in contrast over two-thirds of family physicians were under the age of forty-five (AMA/AAFP 1988: 1278). This generational distinction is reflected in years devoted to postgraduate or residency training. Although many general practice physicians pursued training beyond the required one-year internship, three-year family practice residencies were not formally established until 1970.[3] By 1986, approximately 31 percent of general and family practice physicians had graduated from such programs (AMA/AAFP 1988: 1273–1275). Thus, by the middle of the 1980s, many GPs were moving toward their fourth decade in practice, and their younger competitors were expected to have completed residency training. Historically, physicians in general and family practice provided obstetrical care to patients; as the population of residency-trained physicians grew, the obstetrical competence and hospital privileges of older general practitioners were increasingly challenged and reviewed by "the new guys."

PHYSICIAN DENSITY

Although medically underserved areas exist throughout the country, particularly in rural and impoverished urban areas, the 1980s witnessed a rapid increase in physician density, and it was no longer an anomaly to find board certified internists, pediatricians, and obstetricians as well as family physicians practicing in rural and semirural regions of the country.[4] The sheer increase in the density of primary care clinicians fueled competition in many areas, and the contesting of obstetrical privileges in the language of competence is clearly associated with this overall increase. Regional and historical variations in the practice environment (i.e., whether GPs traditionally practiced obstetrics) as well as the current density of obstetricians in a region influenced whether family physicians continued to provide obstetrical care during the malpractice crises.[5]

THE RESHAPING OF MEDICINE'S
GENDER PROFILE

A dramatic change in medicine over the past two decades has been the extraordinary increase in the proportion of women physicians. A legal and cultural shift, precipitated by the feminist movement's efforts to halt sex bias in public employment and education, and by subsequent antidiscriminatory legislation and the federal funding of medical education in the early 1970s, led to a rapid rise in women admitted to medical schools. In the year 1969/70, 9 percent of first-year students were women; in 1975/76, 20.5 percent; in 1992/93, 41.6 percent of all first-year medical students were women (AAMC/SSS 1992). This remarkable shift has led to a dynamic reconfiguration of the gender profile of the profession, particularly in obstetrics and gynecology.

Although the gender profile of practicing physicians changes more slowly, the number of women in residency programs suggests that the twenty-first century will see quite a different relationship among gender and specialty. No longer restricted to nursing or midwifery, women have sought and been actively recruited to residencies in obstetrics/gynecology in recent years. In 1970, 7.1 percent of OB/GYNs were women; by 1986, 19.6 percent; and by 1990, 22.4 percent, although only 14 percent of board certified OB/GYNs were women in 1992. The change is most notable in the proportion of women in OB/GYN residencies. Prior to 1970 few residents in obstetrics/gynecology—a surgical specialty—were women; in 1975/76, 16.2 percent of first-year residents were women, by 1984, 34 percent, and by 1991/92, 54.1 percent (Roback, Randolph, and Seidman 1992:53–61). A less dramatic increase occurred in family medicine, yet the proportion of women graduates grew from 4.3 percent in 1970 to 12.9 percent in 1986. In 1989, 38 percent of first-year residents in family medicine were women, proportionate to women medical graduates (AMA/AAFP 1988).[6]

This sea change in the gender profile of the profession, and of obstetrics/gynecology and family medicine in particular, may reduce the likelihood that cleavages by gender and specialty will overlap as they did in Coast Community. How this particular transformation in the profession's gender profile will influence debates over obstetrical competence and care remains uncertain.

SPECIALTY BOUNDARIES

Practice boundaries between the primary care specialties of internal medicine, pediatrics, obstetrics, and family medicine have often involved "jurisdictional disputes" (Geyman 1989). As family medicine developed into an academic specialty, one based on residency training rather than on board certification through practice eligibility, turf battles over overlapping practice domains have intensified. These jurisdictional disputes have led to assertions of particular claims to competence, and the development of formal curricula and philosophies of patient care to legitimate these claims (Geyman 1989). Although the "grandfathering in" of the general practitioner to the family medicine specialty through board certification has confounded this effort, the emerging demographic and training profile of the specialty suggests the academic wing of the discipline will carry out future quests for recognized competence.

The Malpractice Crisis and Threats to Obstetrical Care

If the changing demographics of medicine were a significant national development, a second and more readily recognizable force threatening obstetrical practice was the crisis in medical liability. As claim frequencies soared throughout the country for all physicians—from one per thirty-seven physicians in 1968 to one per eight physicians in 1975 and one per five physicians in 1985—obstetricians felt the brunt of the increase, with up to four times as many claims as for internists and family practitioners. In 1985, 73 percent of members surveyed by the American College of Obstetricians and Gynecologists reported at least one claim against them; in 1987, 70.6 percent reported at least one claim. Insurance premiums for obstetricians rose 113 percent between 1982 and 1985 and escalated 238 percent by 1987 (ACOG 1988). In 1985, 18 percent of total practice expenses for OB\GYNs were attributed to medical liability costs; by 1987 these costs had risen even higher to 20.7 percent (Ryan et al. 1989: 4–5; ACOG 1985).

The liability crisis took its toll on the specialty of obstetrics. Twenty-three percent of obstetricians surveyed in 1985 reported they had decreased their high-risk obstetrical care and another 12 percent claimed no longer to offer obstetric care at all (ACOG 1985). ACOG's 1987 survey of members reported a continuation of the attrition cascade, with an additional 12.4 percent withdrawing from obstetrical practice in the previous year (ACOG 1988). Neither age nor generation explained most of the attrition.[7]

Organized obstetrics, through the ACOG, state medical associations, and physician-owned malpractice insurers began to ask why obstetrical claims were more frequent and severe than in other specialties, especially when data did not suggest that adverse outcomes were any higher in obstetrics. Curiously, the initial facile explanation focused on patients' "unrealistic expectations" for "perfect babies" (Jonas 1987; Ryan et al. 1989). A second search for explanation focused on evidence that many obstetrical claims were on behalf of neurologically impaired babies, assumed to be caused by obstetrical events during the course of labor and delivery. In 1985, ACOG estimated that 20 percent of malpractice claims in obstetrics involved the neurologically impaired baby, and other estimates ranged as high as 30 to 40 percent (Ryan et al. 1989; Westbrook and Patchin 1988; ACOG 1988).[8] A third explanation centered on the American legal system and tort law (Ryan et al. 1989; Annandale 1989b). Physicians perceived legislators and lawyers as posing questions not about patients and "unrealistic expectations" or "great disappointments with bad babies" but rather about "bad doctors" and the profession's limitations to assure practice competence (Ryan et al. 1989). (Neurologically impaired babies are referred to as "bad babies" in the idiom of the profession.)

The responses to such questions by ACOG and the political and academic community of obstetrics were impressive. ACOG established a separate department to collect and analyze data on the causes of the malpractice crisis, and to develop strategies to change these liability pressures (AMA/ACOG 1987 [reported in 1988]; ACOG 1985, 1988, 1990). Risk management procedures were reexamined, the process through which standards came to be considered reasonable and appropriate were scrutinized, and the ethics of the locality rule and the role of expert witnesses were reformulated. Research on obstetrical procedures, the birthing process, and causes of infant neurological impairment was encouraged by the discipline, and the academic branch of the specialty reviewed the scientific basis of its knowledge and practice. Curiously, the recent studies on cerebral palsy and intrapartum and obstetrical events threw what had been an assumed certainty of association of asphyxia with cerebral palsy into serious doubt. This effort, although of apparent benefit to the obstetrical community's malpractice defense, created additional ambiguity in standards of practice and judgments of physician competence (Nelson 1988; Nelson and Ellenberg 1984, 1986; Ryan et al. 1989).

Obstetrics also reached out beyond its professional boundaries to relieve liability pressures, with variable success. Public and patient education programs were initiated. And major efforts to reshape policies at the state and national level, in tort reform and in financial coverage for Medicaid patients, were undertaken (AMA/ACOG 1987:3552).

AN ENDANGERED SPECIES?
FAMILY MEDICINE OBSTETRICS

The crisis of the early 1980s that disrupted the specialty of obstetrics soon spilled over to family medicine and nurse-midwifery, as premiums for low-risk obstetrics rose dramatically. Family medicine's own physician attrition from obstetrical practice struck at the heart of the discipline's philosophy of competent comprehensive care, threatening its very domain of practice.[9]

The medical liability environment had a swift and unexpected impact on many family physicians during the critical years 1986–88. The decline in family physicians who practiced hospital obstetrics—from 41 percent in 1985 to 29 percent in 1987—could not simply be attributed to an aging of general practice physicians. Paralleling the rise of liability premiums for low-risk obstetrics and a souring of their feelings about obstetrical practice, physicians fled both the financial and emotional costs of malpractice suits. As illustrated by the Coast Community case, the turmoil of the larger crisis in obstetrics disheartened many physicians on both sides of the specialty divide. For family physicians, the decision not to practice obstetrics appeared less serious than for OB/GYNs. However, the rapid and massive attrition of family physicians from obstetrical practice in the latter half of the 1980s was soon perceived by leaders of the discipline to be greater than first envisioned, a giving up of specialty turf. Accounts of physician "attrition" read like a battle roll. Studies from individual states and national surveys documented dramatic changes; they portray a discipline in crisis, an attrition cascade.

A 1986–87 survey of 464 active members of the AAFP identified 40 percent who had provided obstetrical care in the past and no longer did so. Graduates of residency programs during the 1980s were less likely to begin a practice that included obstetrics than those who had trained prior to 1980. The authors claimed "malpractice issues appeared to play a major role in the decision to discontinue provision of obstetrical services" (Bredfeldt et al. 1989:296).

In California, over half of family physicians who delivered babies in 1985 discontinued doing so in 1986, due ostensibly to the doubling of insurance rates and to the intensification of competition from obstetricians and midwives in many areas (Scherger 1987:95).

In a 1986 survey of 291 members of the Michigan Academy of Family Physicians who had listed themselves as practicing obstetrics, 9.4 percent planned on discontinuing practice in 1987; two-thirds credited liability risk, and over 40 percent mentioned premium costs as the key reason (Smith et al. 1989).

In 1986, graduates of the Alabama-Tuscaloosa Family Practice residency program reported the cost of malpractice insurance was a major cause for dropping obstetrical practice in 1985; those who did so were more likely (92 percent) to have had an obstetrician/gynecologist specialist available within a twenty-five-mile radius, suggesting the importance of competition as well as cost. Seventy-seven percent of all family physicians in the state had provided obstetrical care in the past; in 1981, 56 percent. By 1986 only 13.6 percent of family physicians provided obstetrical care (Tietze et al. 1988).

In 1987, a national survey of 329 family medicine residency graduates identified fear of lawsuits and costs of liability as major reasons for dropping obstetrics, although the density of obstetricians and historical and regional custom were associated causes. Sixty-five percent of respondents had practiced obstetrics at some time; 45 percent were currently practicing obstetrics, although half of these physicians were considering discontinuing obstetrics. Twelve percent had given up obstetrical practice within the past year (Kruse et al. 1989:598). Attrition rates were comparable for all regions of the country.

In 1987, a survey of 282 active members of the Ohio Association of Family Practitioners found a drop in obstetrical practice from 56.7 percent to 21 percent; 16 percent of respondents intended to continue obstetrics into 1989 (Smucker 1988:165–168). The "medicolegal and liability environments" were considered to account for most of the decline. Douglas Smucker found "a dark picture for the survival of obstetrics in family practice in Ohio. The eventual disappearance of all obstetrics practice among family physicians has changed from the unthinkable to a grim possibility" (168).

A 1987 study of eighty-four rural family practice physicians in northern Wisconsin and Minnesota found a somewhat less dismal picture. At the time of the survey, 87 percent of respondents were providing routine obstetrical care, half were providing obstetrical care for high-risk patients, and 23 percent were the primary surgeons for Caesarean sections. Byron Crouse concluded that residency programs needed to continue obstetrical training because "family physicians in rural areas are continuing to be involved actively in providing obstetric care . . . [and] the influence of patient demand and physicians' interest in obstetrics far outweigh the malpractice premium and risk of litigation" (1989:727).

A national survey conducted in 1988 of 3,352 AAFP active members found 28.7 percent held privileges for routine hospital obstetrical care; 11.2 percent also performed complicated deliveries; 12.8 percent performed complicated deliveries "with consultation only." Of these physicians, 38.6 percent did not wish an obstetrical hospital practice and attendant privileges; 18 percent reported liability made the practice of obstetrics prohibitive. In 1980, a similar AAFP survey had found only 5 percent of members reporting a problem with professional liability, and a higher proportion performed complicated deliveries (21 percent) or high-risk obstetrics (15 percent). Rising concern over liability costs and the decline in the practice of obstetrics was regarded by the authors as ominous for the future of the discipline (Schmittling and Tsou 1989:179–184).

Clearly malpractice premiums and fear of litigation were important explanations for family medicine's attrition from obstetrics, but these were the culturally salient and most obvious reasons, current in the litany of physicians' complaints heard throughout the country. In effect, the design of many surveys tapped primarily into this dominant discourse in the profession, producing a response set. Their impact, however, gave the sense of a roll call of practitioners lost in action.

The Response of Academic Family Medicine. In 1987, Joseph Scherger, president of California's organization of family physicians, wondered whether the response of American academic family medicine to the crisis in professional liability was not in fact contributing to "the demise of the family physician who delivered babies" (Scherger 1987). His commentary foretold the chorus of dismay that appeared in subsequent years in the numerous research articles noted above, commentaries, and letters of the AAFP's major journals.[10] Although Scherger argued for a broad analysis that would go beyond attributing attrition solely to professional liability, many articles focused on malpractice costs. By the end of the decade, however, academic family medicine began to address the pragmatics of maintaining obstetrical competence and practice as central to the discipline. Themes of significance for the profession emerged, addressing whether and how family medicine could maintain its position within primary care and offer comprehensive care throughout a family life cycle. By middecade, the very shape of the specialty's practice domain was at stake.

The dismay over attrition from obstetrical practice echoed in the specialty's journals reflects the ideology and contemporary history of family medicine. The academic specialty emerged out of organized general practice, when in 1959 new programs in graduate medical education were first proposed. By 1969, the American Board of Family Practice, the twentieth certification board in American medicine, was established, with a practice-eligible route to diplomate status. By 1970, three-year residency-training programs were launched to meet organized medicine's goal to enhance the status of the general practitioner, a status that had seriously diminished with the rise of the specialties. Family medicine residencies were also designed to provide primary care physicians, particularly for rural areas, in response to political and policy demands (AMA/AAFP 1988:1272–1279). This new specialty was to create a "unique" type of physician, as the formulation of 1975 AAFP Congress of Delegates stated:

The family physician provides health care in the discipline of family practice. His/her training and experience qualify him/her to practice in the several fields of medicine and surgery. The family physician is educated and trained to develop and bring to bear in practice unique attitudes and skills which qualify him or her to provide continuing, comprehensive health maintenance and medical care to the entire family regardless of sex, age or type of problem, be it biological, behavioral or social. This physician serves as the patient's or family's advocate in all health-related matters, including the appropriate use of consultants and community resources. (AMA/AAFP 1988:1273)

Scherger argued that comprehensive care, the "unique" marker of the discipline, would be eroded if family practice physicians were neither adequately trained nor enabled through organizational initiatives to maintain and continue obstetrical practice (Scherger 1987:95).

Others from the field expressed similar concerns, noting "the narrowing of the spectrum of care" (Kruse, Phillips, and Wesley 1989:597), "the abandonment of obstetrics by family physicians," the "deobstetricalization" of family practice (Bredfeldt, Colliver, and Wesley 1989). Some considered that the malpractice issue was but a "scapegoat" and that "obstetrics is too important to be left to the obstetricians" (Klein 1987:167–169). Other faculty pointedly raised the question plaguing the specialty community at large, "Can family physicians practice quality obstetric care and should they?" (Smith 1989:382).

The search for an authorized form of practice, legitimated through research and documented as providing obstetrical competence, colored numerous academic projects of the discipline. At heart were questions about family practice's relationship with the specialty of obstetrics, about practice scope and competency. Could the specialty defend its hard-won practice turf and even promote and expand its domain of low-risk obstetrics?[11] Alternative conceptualizations of obstetrical practice and redefinitions of competence began to emerge in the discipline's research articles, accompanying commentaries, and letters, as the discipline sought to stem the rapid decline of family medicine obstetrics.

Questioning Standards of Practice: The Semantic Domains of Risk

The contemporary discourse on risk, the third major cultural development in medicine, has contributed to the renewed focus on competence, access, and coverage in obstetrical care. High-risk pregnancies and high-risk obstetrics are the domain of obstetrics and gynecology, and defining risk is part of specialty power. The meaning of risk in obstetrics thereby becomes a pivot upon which practice boundaries between obstetrics and family medicine are negotiated. This appears to be a straightforward and uncomplicated empirical endeavor. However, recent queries generated by the malpractice crisis about the meaning of risk have challenged a number of basic assumptions that characterized obstetrics at midcentury and the standards of practice and competence contingent upon these definitions of "risk."[12]

RISK AND OBSTETRICAL COMPETENCE:
A VIEW FROM OBSTETRICS

The American College of Obstetrics and Gynecology in its *Standards for Obstetric-Gynecologic Services* sets forth guidelines, rules, and regulations for organizing obstetrical services in hospital communities. Physician competence in obstetrics is to be based on "education, experience, demonstrated competence, not solely on the basis of board certification" (ACOG 1989:7). A patient's risk factors are assessed in order to provide appropriate management throughout pregnancy and birth. In the sixth edition of the *Standards* (1985), professional privileges are delineated by the "degree of complexity and/ or *risk to patient of condition or illness*" (ACOG [Standards] 1985:8; see table). The *Standards* notes that

Delineation of privileges by category is preferable to other methods. . . . Illness, conditions and procedures are grouped into categories that reflect progressive degrees of patient care complexity, *of risk to the patient,* and of training and experience that the physician needs to manage them. (ACOG [Standards]: 1985:7, 10)

All "high-risk pregnancies including major medical diseases complicating pregnancy except intrauterine transfusions" are considered to be treatable only by a "physician with completed residency training in the specialty or with extensive training or experience in the care of specific conditions" (ACOG [Standards] 1985:8–9).

The specialty of obstetrics/gynecology, therefore, defines its domain of authorized practice, as well as its right to supervise and control the field, through the definition of *risk* and the delineation of physician *competence* required to treat patients in different "at risk" categories. Competence and "risk" are intertwined; high-risk patients require highly skilled, specialty-trained physicians. Competence in risk assessment and patient management is assumed to bear upon the outcomes of pregnancy as well as the procedures required for ensuring "healthy babies and mothers."

SPECIALTY BOUNDARIES AND RISK

Community physicians have traditionally negotiated local practice boundaries between the specialty of obstetrics and family medicine obstetrics. More recently these boundaries have been negotiated at centers of academic medicine, through training programs and research, and through debates over criteria defining high- and low-risk practices, patients, births, and competencies. When obstetricians control local hospital obstetrical privileges, practice boundaries between specialties alter, privileges may be restricted, and competition may circumscribe obstetrical practice by nonspecialists (as illustrated by the case in Coast Community and by the studies summarized above). In general, family physicians have gained privileges for low-risk obstetrics, commensurate with their training and experience, including prenatal care for low-risk patients and uncomplicated vaginal deliveries. A small percentage care for high-risk patients and attend at complicated deliveries, such as breech births or births requiring forceps; far fewer have privileges for Caesarean sections, although some assist surgeons or obstetricians. Use of oxytocin, which may be called for in the dynamics of birthing even for patients initially labeled as low-risk, appears to be an area of contention among the specialties.

The broad policies on obstetrical practice, utilizing a categorical approach to defining levels of risk and physician competencies required to attend to patients at each level, are clearly defined by ACOG and generally accepted by the American Board of Family Practice. Both agree on the necessity of assessing the risk status of patients and of requiring demonstrated physician competence and appropriate training. Nevertheless, the definitional process through which an originally low-risk patient becomes a high-risk patient frequently depends on the perspective of the clinician and may be less clear than categorical definitions imply. Such ambiguity heightens tension between the specialties, as redesignation into a high-risk category may lead to a complicated delivery, with the expectation of referral to an obstetrician. That this process of assessing risk is fraught with uncertainty is documented in the complaints of family physicians and obstetricians about each others' practices (LeFevre, Williamson, and Hector 1989; Sayres 1989; Scherger 1988; Wall 1988; Wall et al. 1989; see also chapter 4).

RISK ASSESSMENT: A VIEW
FROM FAMILY MEDICINE

In the late 1980s, family medicine academics, recognizing the pivotal importance of the definition of high-risk patients as well as high-risk obstetrics for the discipline's future in obstetrical care, began to explore risk assessment scoring systems. Such systems, it was hoped, would document in a "scientifically" acceptable fashion (i.e., with statistical and epidemiological documentation) those patients who would legitimately fall within the family medicine domain of authorized practice. In the search for certainty, the academics uncovered ambiguity.

In 1988 and 1989, the *Journal of Family Practice* published several articles on obstetrics risk assessment and outcome. In an evaluation of risk scoring systems for adverse outcomes of pregnancy, Eric Wall concluded:

Risk-scoring systems are frequently used to predict perinatal outcomes and anticipated health care needs. They have determined which patients received care from which type of provider, which patients deliver in a birthing room as opposed to a delivery suite, and in some settings, which patients are candidates for a home birth. It should be obvious that a risk-scoring system that may be helpful in one area is not automatically useful for another very different kind of decision. (1988:156)

Researchers turned toward population-based studies and clinical epidemiology to search for certainty (LeFevre, Williamson, and Hector 1989; Sayres 1989; Wall et al. 1989). In subsequent analyses of patients for whom risk scores were calculated, they found that while most scoring systems were helpful in identifying clinically problematic situations, they were less useful in their positive predictive value of high-risk outcomes. This lack of certainty led Michael LeFevre and his colleagues to summarize that

the majority of adverse outcomes will occur in women identified as low risk. The risk-scoring system in this population was no more effective than a policy that would refer all women with standard obstetric risk factors. (LeFevre, Williamson, and Hector 1989:691)

William Sayres, from the University of Utah family medicine faculty, noted a *negligible* correlation between the risk score and pregnancy and birth outcomes of 309 patients, concluding the system was "poorly predictive." In addition, low socioeconomic status, usually considered a risk factor for poor birth outcomes "was found to be *significantly* . . . associated with better rather than worse outcome" (1989:266–267).

These findings had medicolegal as well as territorial ramifications. In a commentary, Scherger noted that "current risking systems are vitally important to the family physician, if only for their dreaded medicolegal implications," and "family physicians must be active in the dialogue" on risk assessment "to preserve their role in this critically important area of family practice" (1988:162–163). Sayres, noting that the risk-scoring system in use in the Utah practice was urged as a referral guideline by their major insurer, commented that "the medicolegal tail is wagging the family practice dog."

The ambiguity over risk assessment stirred certain fears among the family medicine community—as evidenced in both letters and commentaries in the *Journal of Family Practice*. If low-risk patients ended up with high-risk outcomes—"risking out," premature birthing, low-birth-weight infants in need of perinatal high-tech care—could family medicine realistically claim any low-risk patient care as their own? Faculty response was astute and political. In a commentary on Wall's 1988 article on the usefulness and limits of risk assessment and scoring systems, Scherger argued for an approach that would broaden rather than restrict academic family medicine's role, noting that the review "puts formal obstetric risk-scoring mechanisms in perspective by showing that all are imprecise and may not be better than good clinical judgment." He argued that

Family Practice has a vested interest in taking a leadership role in the determination of risk in pregnancy and the development of practice standards. . . . A practical interpretation . . . requires a clear separation of two issues: the identification of risk in pregnancy and the issue of formal scoring mechanisms to determine quantitatively the risk. . . . What is important for the physician in practice is not which mechanism is used to quantify the risk status of a patient but whether the physician is *equipped* to recognize and manage risk when it is present. (Scherger 1988:162–163)

Calling for a "new direction in family practice maternity care," away from the "mini-obstetrician," currently salient in family medicine, Scherger argued that all pregnancies and births should be assumed to be natural and low-risk unless otherwise demonstrated (1988:163). This astute analysis identified how risk assessment and clinical competence are intertwined and acknowledged the medicolegal and specialty politics embedded in the intertwining.

THE MEANING OF "RISK MANAGEMENT"

"Risk management" gives the meaning of "risk" an ironic twist. Acknowledging that the patient's risk becomes the physician's risk, risk management programs seek to reduce the likelihood of medical accidents, patient harm, and malpractice claims. By the late 1980s, numerous programs were developed by organized groups within the specialties of obstetrics/gynecology and family medicine. In addition, insurers, hospitals, and residency training programs began to seek solutions to the malpractice crisis. Risk management activities were not confined to individual physicians or to clinical practice. Rather, programs were political and legal as well as medical and scientific, as state legislatures, Congress, health policymakers, and lawyers became involved.[13]

Risk management efforts were variously defined. An obstetrician offered the following suggestions at the medical malpractice symposium held in 1987 at Harvard:

identification of poor practice; proper reactions to that in the form of eliminating deficiencies or restricting practice; . . . and the study of causation of disease—so that when something happens whose cause is genuinely not understood, it is not automatically attributed to bad practice. (Fredric D. Frigoletto, in Ryan et al. 1989:10)

In family medicine, risk management programs were initiated with the goal of enhancing obstetrical competence through continuing education and chart review. Programs emphasized standardizing records and review of physician practice in "perinatal risk assessment, appropriate consultation and referral, as well as appropriate prenatal, labor and delivery management" (Scherger and Tanji 1987:12–13).[14]

Educational programs were proposed to "include patients in the uncertainties of medical practice" (AMA/ACOG 1987; Ryan et al. 1989; Annandale 1989a), and a renewed look at informed consent procedures was undertaken. In addition, physicians were urged to develop good relationships with patients, to "Communicate, Communicate, Communicate" (Annandale 1989a), the assumption being that patients who have good relationships with their physicians are less likely to sue. Thus, as the profession sought ways to stem the rise in malpractice claims, patient-physician relationships were reexamined.

RISK MANAGEMENT VIA SCIENTIFIC
RESEARCH: SHATTERING "CLINICAL MYTHS"

From 1987 through 1990, two major "clinical myths" that had guided obstetrical practice and the assessment of competence and culpability in malpractice were critically reviewed by the scientific community (IOM 1989b:1057–1060; AMA/ACOG 1987; Ryan et al. 1989). The first assumption, held since clinical descriptions of the phenomena appeared in the nineteenth century, associated cerebral palsy with perinatal events marked by meconium in the amniotic fluid or by bradycardia, both considered to be indicative of intrapartum asphyxia. The second was the highly conventional practice that allowed physicians to identify these indicative conditions through the technology of electronic fetal monitoring.

Electronic fetal monitoring and its benefits had been debated throughout the 1970s and 1980s and continue to be questioned today. William Arney, in an excellent analysis of the place of electronic fetal monitoring in contemporary obstetrics (1982), reviewed the scientific literature on EFM (electronic fetal monitoring) published from 1968 to 1978. He contends that the continued and widespread use of electronic fetal monitoring in American obstetrics, despite ambiguous findings as to its benefits, was part of the discipline's movement toward wider surveillance and monitoring of pregnancy, labor, and birth. The discrepancy between clinical practice, clinical sense, and clinical science appears less odd when placed within these broad historical developments in the specialty (Arney 1982:99–154). Despite the lack of unambiguous favorable scientific findings, electronic fetal monitoring has been a standard of practice in American obstetrics into the early 1990s. An Institute of Medicine study on professional liability and obstetrical care argued that Americans had adopted electronic fetal monitoring "as standard practice, at considerable added expense to routine obstetrical care, despite the failure of scientific evidence to support its use" (IOM 1989b:1058).

In March of 1990, a study published in the *New England Journal of Medicine* presented the disturbing findings that premature infants monitored with electronic fetal monitoring had *higher* odds (2.9) for having cerebral palsy than did a comparable group of infants who were monitored externally, by periodic auscultation (Shy et al. 1990: 588–593). These findings and assessments such as the IOM review suggest an uncertain future for this deeply entrenched routine technological practice.

The assumed link between intrapartum distress and cerebral palsy was also reexamined. This "clinical myth," an essential part of obstetrical knowledge, had guided decisions on Caesarean sections and produced technological innovations for intervention in the natural process of birth. It was also knowledge used to judge physician performance in response to signs of fetal distress. Given that a very high proportion of malpractice claims are on behalf of neurologically impaired babies, this clinical knowledge was powerful in establishing traditions of obstetrical practice.

Epidemiological studies by National Institutes of Health neurologist

Karin Nelson, reported at the Harvard symposium on malpractice and obstetrics, asked, How much cerebral palsy can be related to obstetric events, in particular to preventable obstetric events? The researchers found the unexpected—a "surprisingly" weak association between cerebral palsy and intrapartum events, such as the presence of meconium and bradycardia (Nelson, in Ryan et al. 1989:53–61; see also Nelson 1988 and Nelson and Ellenberg 1986).[15] Nelson's talk, "Shattering the Clinical Myths," highlighted what she referred to as the "irrationality in the system" of judging obstetrical competence in malpractice cases (Ryan et al. 1989:61). Nelson's findings are relevant to how the medical profession responded politically to the malpractice crisis. Dr. Julius Richmond,[16] long engaged in policymaking, commented upon the importance of the findings:

The knowledge base has changed. . . . The old notions about what caused cerebral palsy, largely promulgated when Dr. Little presented his first descriptions in the [nineteenth] century, became so deeply embedded that it's very difficult to get them out of the system. . . . [It] would be a serious error for us to underestimate the importance of the shift in the knowledge base. . . . [Nelson and colleagues] have taken modern epidemiology and brought us really new insights into causation [and] have shown how few of our past notions about causation really were valid. (Richmond, quoted in Ryan et al. 1989:66)

Another physician panelist, James Mongan, regarded Nelson's findings as the "key difference between malpractice in obstetrics and malpractice in other specialties," noting that what

data show us is that there is absolutely no genuine and reliable scientific data base upon which these decisions are now being adjudicated. We have heard lawyers say it's totally arbitrary, close to totally arbitrary, or very arbitrary. My own strong plea is that if, indeed, we are dealing with something that's nearly a random crap-shoot, we should do our very best to develop an alternative system for this class of cases. I think we have that obligation—to do something better than just wait around for 10 or 15 years, and let this terribly arbitrary, unscientific, and unfair system go on. Why? Because there's more than an economic cost here. There are emotional costs as well, and other costs, too. . . . [and] we have an obligation to try and do better than simply wait for knowledge to trickle down. (Ryan et al. 1989:67)

Curiously, Nelson's findings, incorporated into the Institute of Medicine's report on professional liability and obstetrical care (IOM 1989a), had been published in the major medical journals several years prior to the Harvard symposium and the IOM review (Nelson and Ellenberg 1984, 1986; Nelson 1988). Did it necessitate a conference and an IOM report to crystallize the impact of this scientific research or was it possibly tainted, appearing "self-serving" and a "conflict of interest" on the part of the specialty of obstetrics? (Robertson 1988:362).

What explains the delay in professional response? A clear explanation is not obvious, although the culture and political economies of obstetrical practice may complicate the incorporation of new knowledge into the specialty's science.[17] Nevertheless, the continuing negative assessments of electronic fetal monitoring and knowledge questioning the link between obstetrical practice and cerebral palsy influenced the meanings of risk and of competent care. What was implied by the "standards of care" by which physicians had been judged and evaluated in malpractice cases, and in which they had been trained?

RISK AND ACCESS: FLEEING FROM RISK AND "ECONOMICALLY AT RISK" PATIENTS

Although the response of organized and academic medicine to the malpractice crisis was aimed at preserving obstetrical practice, individual physicians took more direct steps to limit their risk of suit. Not only did many physicians stop delivering babies, numerous others restricted care for patients deemed to be "high risk." Spontaneous efforts by individual physicians to limit high-risk obstetrics affected low-income patients most severely. Sixty percent of all state Medicaid programs and 90 percent of all Maternal and Child Health programs were having difficulty recruiting providers (IOM 1989b). The threat of a malpractice suit and low reimbursement of Medicaid (often lower than the per-patient cost for malpractice premiums) were considered chief causes. The IOM report noted the same problems had affected the "organization and practice of nurse-midwifery" (1989b:1058). In addition, the IOM attributed to physicians an *unsubstantiated* yet widely prevalent assumption that "the poor were more litigious than the middle and upper classes" and thus more likely to put them "at risk" of suit (IOM 1989b:1058).[18] As physicians fled risk of suit, access to quality care became ever more difficult for those "economically at risk": the rural patient, the poor patient, the Medicaid patient, the patient without insurance.

The Irony of Specialty Boundaries. The practical consequences of physicians fleeing high-risk patients unfolded as the malpractice crisis intensified. Patients, in particular high-risk patients in

rural areas, encountered barriers to care from specialty high-risk obstetricians and were compelled to seek obstetrical care from general
practitioners. The irony of this trend, especially in the context of the
academic debate over what kind of practitioner should provide obstetrical care and to whom, is powerful.[19]

The literature documents the passing of Medicaid or uninsured patients to those lower in the hierarchy of obstetrical power and expertise: to midwives (Annandale 1989a) and to family or general practice
physicians (IOM 1989a; Onion and Mockapetris 1988). However, restricting or withholding care from economically "at-risk" patients was
not simply motivated by individual quirks. In some states and communities, as in Coast Community, physicians used their services as political leverage, deliberately provoking a public crisis, to gain more
remuneration for care provided to Medicaid patients and to prompt
legislators to pass tort and malpractice reform. The poor suffered the
most from these efforts.[20] Letters and commentaries in professional
journals and at malpractice conferences indicate physician awareness of
the political motivations behind such actions. Nevertheless, such actions were in themselves "risky," often jeopardizing the public trust,
and patients, physicians, and the public often experienced the negative
consequences that arose from withholding obstetrical services.

CONTROLLING UNCERTAINTY AND
THE MEANING OF RISK

Through efforts to define and control risk, both in terms
of physician practice and patient characteristics, the disciplines of ob-
stetrics/gynecology and family medicine sought to enhance certainty,
to promote rationality. Our popular culture's conceptualization of
birth as a natural process and the high rate of normal outcomes and
"well" babies defy any easy acknowledgment of uncertainty, either by
physicians, patients, or the public. Yet the enormous pain experienced
by families, physicians, and all care providers when babies do not survive or are seriously impaired grants gravity to the drive for certainty
and control. The malpractice crisis in obstetrics disrupted widely held
assumptions about the certainty of standards of practice, scientific and
clinical knowledge, and evaluations of physician competence. However, many efforts to effect certainty and to control uncertainty, through
the development of risk-scoring systems and risk management projects
and through reexamination of the scientific knowledge base of clinical

practice and evaluations of professional work, led to greater ambiguity, to increasing uncertainty. These efforts revealed a fundamental uncertainty in clinical practice.

Philosophies of Birthing and Professional Boundaries

The fourth major cultural development against which the crisis in obstetrical care continues to unfold has been a flourishing of competing philosophies of birthing. Debates over ideal obstetrical care and modes of birthing, carried forth in both lay and professional settings, continue to contribute to the discourse on competition and competence among the specialties of obstetrics, family medicine, and midwifery. The following interpretations of the medical specialties' philosophies—indeed, ideologies—of birthing are but partial; however, they represent diverse voices in medicine today and the audiences to which they direct their case for competence in obstetrical care. Although the substance of debates over obstetrical care focuses on modes of birthing and questions of intervention and use of technology, the debates are also about professional power and hierarchy. Whereas the specialty of obstetrics looks to its medical and surgical traditions, to the women's health movement, and to its potential patients in presenting its case on birthing and practice, family medicine appears compelled to compare its philosophy to that of the specialty of obstetrics to distinguish family medicine from those who ultimately dominate the field—the obstetricians. The following "points of view" are drawn from the literature published by each discipline.

A VIEW FROM FAMILY MEDICINE

The current dominant ideology of family practice obstetrics emphasizes a low-technology/low-intervention approach to obstetrical care as exemplified by its position on "risk" and training reviewed thus far. This low-risk, low-technology, low-intervention, and "high-touch" hallmark serves to protect the discipline's practice domain. It also provides family medicine with a clear ideological divide between itself and the specialty of obstetrics in terms of technology and "risk," in effect placing the specialty on the side popularly regarded as "the good," connecting physicians with American cultural movements on low-intervention birthing. Leaders in the discipline argue that to compare the obstetrical competence and outcomes of family physicians with those of obstetricians fails to acknowledge the "unique" emphasis of family practice (which is similar to that of midwifery). And they contend that such comparisons diminish the consistently demonstrated positive outcomes of the low-intervention approach for low-risk patients (Brody and Howe 1987; Klein et al. 1992; Rosenblatt 1988; Scherger 1987, 1988; Smith, Green, and Schwenk 1988).

Asserting the philosophy of low-intervention birthing care has curricular and political implications for family medicine. If the high technology of specialty obstetrics is eschewed, and the preferred path to training and competence is not to emulate the specialty through the creation of mini-obstetricians, then judgments of physician obstetrical competence may reside at least in part within the boundaries of family medicine.

Despite this ideology of practice and goals to control training, the definition of obstetrical competence for family physicians continues to be framed in terms of standards established by the specialty of obstetrics. The refrain prevailing in much of the literature compares family physicians with obstetricians (Bowman 1989; Kriebel and Pitts 1988; Mengel and Phillips 1987; Ornstein et al. 1990; Rosenblatt 1988).

Are we as family physicians as competent as the obstetricians in providing quality obstetrical care?

Are we as capable or competently trained in the mastery of the prevailing technology in the field (ultrasound being the most recently examined)?

Are we as competent at exercising judgment (risk scoring and clinical risk assessment)?

Can we manage difficult situations that emerge in the dynamics of pregnancy and delivery (managing low-birth-weight infants)?

Why assume that standards of care set by specialists are appropriate for generalists as well?

Against the comparative refrain, other voices from within family medicine echo those from midwifery, the women's health movement, and patients: high technology and interventionist approaches to birthing are not necessarily beneficial and seldom desirable for patients.

They pose questions:.

Are family physicians uncritically adopting the obstetricians' practice style? (Brody 1987:242)

Are different paradigms needed in family practice, not only to stop the "relentless increase in the technologizing of obstetrics" but also to preserve, in the face of attrition and the medical liability crisis, obstetrical practice in family medicine for the decade of the 1990s? (Rosenblatt 1988:128–129)

Should not family medicine encourage research on the "appropriate application of technology" in primary care obstetrics "in hopes of preventing iatrogenic morbidity caused by unlimited use of interventions with inherent risks to emotional and physical health"? (Smith, Green, and Schwenk, 1989:383)

"In spite of the competition from obstetrical specialists, should not family practice consider filling the void left by the attrition of obstetricians, especially in rural and underserved urban areas?" (Rakel 1989:2846)

For family medicine, espousing a philosophy of low-intervention birthing justifies the discipline's practice "turf and territory."[21]
Efforts at the state and federal political level, among insurers, and in academic settings where the discipline struggles to preserve obstetrical practice *and* training are colored by these concerns. And because the obstetrical community has begun to question the knowledge base of standards of practice and therefore standards for judgment of provider competence, family medicine's struggles have acquired a particularly interesting cast. If standards such as the use of electronic fetal monitoring are no longer assumed to be the obvious practice of choice, then which discipline's philosophy of obstetrics is to be used to judge physician competence, to establish and control training curricula, and to assess negligence in malpractice suits?

A VIEW FROM OBSTETRICS

The women's health movement has been central to transformations in obstetrical ideology and the philosophy of birthing for over two decades, and yet the movement's influence on the specialty of obstetrics is complex. Recent feminist literature and women's personal accounts critically view the alienating features of contemporary obstetrics (Davis-Floyd 1992; Martin 1987), pointing to the hegemonic technologies of clinical practice. In contrast, Arney argues that since 1945, the specialty of obstetrics has been in dialogue with its consumers (he refers to this as "a univocal discourse between modern women and modern obstetrics"), readily introducing natural childbirth and accommodating women's interest in psychological satisfaction into considerations of practice (Arney 1982). Both interpretations hold merit. The specialty of obstetrics continues to monitor its potential patients, the women's health movement, and its competitors—family medicine physicians and midwives—with the explicit intent to maintain control of the field. Certainly the introduction of birthing centers and family-centered maternity care are among the notable innovations in marketing obstetrical care in the last quarter of the twentieth century that the specialty had advanced and—when in control—supported.[22]

Harry Jonas, a former head of ACOG, commenting on the AMA's *Council Report: The Future of Obstetrics/Gynecology*, assessed the influence of the women's health movement on the profession in a more jaded vein. Under the title "The Torch Is Passed" he noted that this once "happy field of medicine" has "experienced more dramatic and radical changes than any other medical specialty" and stated that it is the patient who "plunges the obstetrician-gynecologist into the briar patch of controversy." He lamented that "gone is . . . the easy ambience of the past when a woman's 'OB' was at most a god, and at least, a father figure" (Jonas 1987:3554).

The source of the dramatic reshaping of practice in obstetrics and gynecology, Jonas argues, is the women's health movement and the specialty's focus on "how, to whom and by whom" health care is to be provided. He suggests the *Council Report* underemphasizes the importance of

the consumer health movement in altering change of practice patterns, in large part fueled by the feminist movement. Women, throughout history, have sought, and, lately, demanded a voice in how women's health care services are provided to them. Consider how patients have influenced such medical practices as the use of episiotomy, obstetrical forceps and caesarean section. The manner and location in which labor and delivery are conducted, the use or nonuse of pain relief in deliveries, and even whether labor and delivery are conducted with the patient supine or upright all demand a special type of physician-patient relationship in which the patient participates actively and significantly in the management of her medical care. (1987:3555)

Despite these developments in the discourse between women and the profession, low-intervention birthing still eludes many patients. The use of diagnostic technology, electronic fetal monitoring, and Caesarean sections increased steadily throughout the 1980s and into the 1990s (AMA/ACOG 1987:3551). The use of technology during pregnancy and birth was not significantly precluded by the influence of either the women's movement or contemporary ideologies of appropriate birthing experiences. Curiously, Caesarean sections were somewhat "detechnologized" during the 1980s (or as consumers became more comfortable with medical techniques, there was a "normalizing" of Caesarean births), as husbands were allowed in the delivery theater and local anesthesia was used, to enhance the "birthing experience" of women and the bonding of mother and child.[23] Concomitant changes—increased use of reproductive technologies, extended monitoring during pregnancy and birthing, the rise in rate of Caesarean sections, and the incorporation of interests of patients and the women's movement—were not necessarily nor always in contradiction.

Although the specialty of obstetrics presents low-intervention philosophies of birthing for public consumption and marketing, the criteria required for a woman to become a legitimate candidate for a low-intervention birth are still contested. The specialty views itself as having the privilege, indeed the expertise and the authority, to set these criteria. Recall the comment by the family practice professor who remarked that "a woman has to be 'bionic' to make it into the obstetricians' low-risk category!" Low-intervention approaches to obstetrical care are tolerated or even encouraged by obstetricians, many of whom hire midwives to attend normal vaginal deliveries. Yet because the boundaries between low- and high-risk patients and situations are ambiguous, and in fact have been blurred by the very technology designed to establish certainty, the creation of distinctions of risk is inherently problematic. This is particularly true during the dynamic course of labor when women might "risk out."

Alternative birthing practices continue to be enthusiastically espoused by many obstetricians who are especially attuned to the contemporary popular culture of birthing and to consumer economics. Others view alternative practices as marginal to the essence of this surgical-medical specialty. In residency training, when competence in high-technology, high-risk, and surgical obstetrics is taught and emphasized, low-intervention birthing is also taught, but primary responsibility for patient care is often shared or passed on to other members of the obstetrical team, to midwives, and even to medical students who are lower in the hierarchy of power and surgical expertise. In the context of academic medicine and in health politics, low-intervention approaches may be extolled, but research demonstrating that birthing centers are as "competent" and successful as obstetrical units in producing good outcomes for low-risk births continues to be debated (Annandale 1989a; Rooks et al. 1989).

Yet the influence of the women's health movement and the changing demographic profile of women patients and of obstetricians have been acknowledged by those who speak for the specialty as critical to their specialty's competitive edge. The *Council Report* concluded:

The most salient issues for the specialty in the future [are] . . . (1) the direction of the professional liability crisis, (2) medical practice competition, (3) the feminization of poverty, (4) ethical issues arising from technological and social imperatives, (5) the changing gender profile of the specialty, and (6) the impact of the feminist movement on women's health care. (AMA/ACOG 1987:3547)

The *Council Report*'s assessment of the influence of concerns about cost containment and the women's health movement led to a prediction that intensive-care birth settings would be common in the 1990s. These developments have materialized in many obstetrical units, as the specialty responded to market competition, to popular desire for "psychological satisfaction with birthing," and to pressures from health maintenance organizations for cost containment. The specialty also monitors its competition from family medicine and midwifery, and has redefined its image to range from high-technology expertise to primary care obstetrics and social gynecology.[24]

True to the specialty's essential identity, however, the focus on technology is diffused throughout the *Council Report*'s predictions and planning for its future. Technological expertise and innovations are not only envisioned but justified in terms of cost containment, and new diagnostic technology is linked to the future enhancement and expansion of alternative birthing programs. And women who have delayed pregnancy until their thirties are considered new territory for an "increase in the use of other services for obstetric patients, such as . . . ultrasonography, amniocentesis, and fetal monitoring" (AMA/ACOG 1987:3550).

A Turning Point in Obstetrical Care?

Is there a turning point in obstetrical practice and care emerging from the tumultuous decade of the 1980s? The demographic changes in women who seek obstetrical care, the professional and public responses to the medical liability and malpractice crisis in obstetrics, and the changing gender profile of the specialty of obstetrics suggest that the practice of modern obstetrics reached a turning point in the 1990s.

Jonas, commenting on the AMA council's report on obstetrics in "Passing the Torch," challenges the new women obstetricians—neither "father figure" nor "god" to their patients—to redress the crisis in obstetrics and assure the future:

The feminist movement helped to kick off a part of this upheaval in the specialty. Now it seems that women will be in the forefront of meeting these challenges. . . . The feminization of the specialty *will* have an impact on practice patterns and possibly on medical decision making. It will undoubtedly move us well beyond the "doctor knows best" era. Whatever our gender, we must *learn to listen* to what the patient is saying. (Jonas 1987:3555)

Whatever the specialty, the health of obstetrical care and obstetrical providers may also depend on what "the patient is saying."

JOINING FORCES

At the national and state level, collaboration and dialogue between the specialties of obstetrics/gynecology and family medicine continue to be difficult. Competition for patients and economic viability and disputes over philosophies of birthing and the meaning of professional competence will continue to affect this relationship. Yet the call to develop common remedies to redress practices that harm patients and lead to malpractice claims (risk management) illustrates the political sensibility of the profession. The professional literature acknowledges the ingrained competition between the two disciplines; responses have been prescriptive and somewhat cautious. Although competition between family medicine and obstetrics will shape the future of both specialties, the need to "improve the dialogue" and to "strengthen liaison efforts" is considered of paramount importance by both, in particular if actions to affect public policies on "liability pressures" are to meet with success.[25] This call to join forces to frame the future of obstetrical care for the next century represents a contemporary effort by medicine seeking to assert control where ambiguity lies.

There is an uncanny parallel between what happened to obstetrical practice and care in Coast Community and the events that unfolded on a national scale during the same period in our country's "obstetrical" history. One of the most striking parallels was the mixing of "risk talk," in all its ambiguity, with the discourse on professional competence. In the community context, the mixing of "risk-competence" talk produced an increasingly heated colloquial commentary on obstetrical competence and provider legitimacy, on hierarchy and power, on practice boundaries between specialties, and on medical malpractice. The competence-risk discourse of the coast's physicians was not only directed to other physicians and professionals such as the midwives and hospital administrators but it engaged patients and the general public as well. Thus, conflicting ideologies of birthing and gender competition and fears of malpractice were articulated in terms of risk and competence at public meetings and in the media as well as in professional circles. At the national level, in medical research literature, in published clinical standards and guidelines, and in essays and letters of clinicians, the discourse on risk and competence articulated similar concerns: How could the malpractice crisis be contained and resolved? What constituted authorized practice and knowledge? Who should control obstetrical practice and care? Ultimately, the risk-competence discourse, even in formal repertoire, spoke to specialty hierarchy and power and to competition over the obstetrical domain. Yet, at both the national and local levels, the risk-competence discourse is also about mastering uncertainty in obstetrical practice, about reducing harm to patients and improving patient care, and about improving the competence of physicians who deliver that care.

The Quest for Competence through Medical Education

Introduction to Part II

Curricular innovation is ubiquitous in American medical education, reflecting in part dynamic transformations in biomedical knowledge and techniques and in part the political economy of how that knowledge is produced and taught. Curricular innovations also institutionalize continuous deliberations by medical faculties about what constitutes medical competence and how students need to be educated and socialized into the profession. In this section, I explore a facet of the puzzle on the meaning of physician competence which seeks the source of its symbolic and existential power for individual physicians and for the profession of medicine as a whole, and turn to examine social practices and discursive interactions in medical training that make competence the essence of professional achievement and identity.

My ethnographic text grows out of a study of curricular innovation at Harvard Medical School, initially known as the New Pathway, which my husband and I carried out during the program's introduction and institutionalization (1986–1991).[1] We began the study in the second year of the experimental curriculum, when 38 of 160 students in the incoming class of 1990 were selected to pursue the New Pathway. We interviewed students from each curriculum, from the classes of 1989, 1990, and 1991, and followed a cohort systematically through their preclinical and clinical training.[2] We participated in tutorials and classes; attended curriculum meetings and workshops where educational innovations were debated, devised, and revised; interviewed faculty and administrators who were involved in creating the New Pathway, as well as those who were skeptical or opposed; and taught in both the traditional and New Pathway curricula.

Harvard was not the first medical school in North America to introduce self-directed learning and problem-based tutorials in the basic sciences, accompanied by early clinical training. McMaster University Medical School was founded on these educational innovations, in 1966.[3] Nor was Harvard the first to replace a "proven" lecture-based curriculum with case-based tutorials often taught by generalists rather than experts. The University of New Mexico experimented with a student-directed and tutorial-based curriculum in parallel with a traditional curriculum for over ten years, before generalizing and revising it for all students in 1993. However, the Harvard "experiment" was highly visible, drawing national attention not only from other medical schools but from the popular media as well.[4]

Under the leadership of a visionary dean and his faculty supporters, a new ethos and, in a very tangible sense, a new culture legitimizing experimentation and innovation were quickly institutionalized, as the "New Pathway" of 1985 became the "Common Pathway" for all students who matriculated in 1987. Nevertheless, an ardent debate over what would constitute the school's educational ethos, its essential "cultural" image, colored the early years of innovation during which the majority of students from the 1989 and 1990 classes followed the "classic curriculum" and, in the opinion of many faculty, the "proven pathway" to medical competence. Resistance to the innovation appeared most entrenched at the teaching hospitals, where some residents and faculty questioned the case-based tutorials and other innovations in basic science teaching and expressed vocal skepticism about the competence of their new "clerks." Efforts to redesign clinical training in the spirit of the New Pathway met resistance, despite the initiation of ambulatory clerkships and a third-year "patient-doctor" tutorial. Recognizing that effective transformation of the culture and ethos of clinical training required aggressive persistence, one dean remarked that he worried that "the New Pathway is a wave that crashes on the shores of the clerkships."[5]

Renee Fox, writing about the new medical curricula of earlier decades, observed:

The new curriculum is premised on the notion that medical education not only affects the outlook and comportment of individual physicians, but also the attributes of the profession and the larger system of which doctors are a part. (Fox 1988:95)

Her 1974 essay "Is There a 'New' Medical Student? A Comparative View of Medical Socialization in the 1950s and the 1970s" (included in Fox 1988) places the new wave of curricular innovations in historical continuity.[6] Fox suggested that the medical educators of the 1970s had high "socialization consciousness" (1988:95), perhaps influenced by studies of professional socialization carried out in the 1950s by Chicago and Columbia sociologists (Becker et al. 1961; Merton, Reader, and Kendall 1957). Similar assessments could be made of leading medical educators today. The changes of the 1970s—from early contact with patients from all social classes to courses on ethics "to ponder death and dying and the moral implications . . . of biomedical advances"— were the "organized attempts" of educators to meet "the criticism and self-criticism to which the American medical profession and health care system have been subject in recent years" (Fox 1988:94).

These interpretations resonate with contemporary efforts to reform medical education in the 1990s, to create physicians for the twenty-first century.[7] However, at the *fin-de-siècle*, "the new biology" and the extraordinary proliferation of medical knowledge and techniques drive innovations in how the sciences basic to medicine are organized and taught. Critical discussions by medical faculties about how best to teach the new biology and the new genetics bear upon how schools politically organize education in the biosciences and clinical training. Underlying these efforts, and the struggles to control the direction of innovation and change, is the fundamental goal of educating future doctors who can competently integrate the new sciences and technology into humane patient care.[8]

The next two chapters focus on student experiences of medical education in the clinical training years. I explore how students learn increasingly complex narrative strategies for presenting medically relevant data (chapter 6) and acquire clinical competence and responsibility for patient care through interacting and identifying with the clinical training hierarchy (chapter 7). Throughout these training experiences, students discover and internalize the subtleties of the meaning of competence and its uses in medical work and medical politics. They learn medicine's multiple discourses on competence and the contexts in which they are encouraged, condoned, or negatively sanctioned. This process of discovery and internalization makes competence fundamental to the everyday clinical work and professional experience of American physicians, creating a dimension of its social reality. Given that discourses on medical competence characterize moments of educational innovation, I begin my ethnographic account with a recollection of the early debates about the New Pathway, thereby setting the stage for student experience.

CHAPTER SIX

Narrative Strategies in Presentation and Performance

From Artifice to Competence

I want to know what we're going to be competent at. What does Harvard expect of us? They don't really tell us!
—First-year student, class of 1990

Nobody could find it in their hearts to let me, and many of us, know that things were working. . . . I walked out of [first year] not knowing anything.
—Third-year New Pathway student

Institutionalizing the Experimental: The New Pathway

Sweeping changes in medical education constituted the agenda for the decade of the 1980s at Harvard Medical School. The New Pathway, an innovative and "experimental" curriculum, was introduced to a largely skeptical faculty and eager but anxious student body in 1985. Although offered as an experiment by the deans of the Medical School (Deans Daniel Tosteson, S. James Adelstein, and Daniel Federman, and Harvard's President Derek Bok), the innovations embodied a wholesale critique of traditional lecture-based approaches to medical education.[1] These critiques, by implication, included the preclinical courses taught by nearly all of the medical school's basic science faculty. In the early years of the experiment, as the New Pathway curriculum evolved, distinctions between the traditional and the experimental curriculums were often linked to deep and irrational metaphors in American medical culture. The innovators juxtaposed the "active" or problem-based learning of New Pathway basic science tutorials over against the lectures of the traditional curriculum, which by default became caricatured as "passive" learning. Basic science faculty opposed to the innovation, offended by the active/passive metaphors, commented on "the lack of content at the expense of process," on "the lack of expertise," the "endless conversations" about what students did not know. And they criticized the teaching of basic science by "generalists" or clinicians without basic science degrees, perhaps masking resistance to the new interdisciplinary courses. Such discussions continued even after all students matriculated, in 1987, in the Common/New Pathway.

The traditional and new curricula were also juxtaposed in terms of humanism or "caring." The New Pathway was promoted (and interpreted in the media) as committed to the ideals of improving relationships between patients and physicians, and experimental tutorials led by clinicians exposed students to early patient contact, training in clinical skills and psychosocial assessment, and discussions of critical issues in the patient-doctor relationship. Ethics, social science, and psychosocial knowledge were reframed and taught—largely by clinicians—through the patient-doctor case-based tutorials. The popular media seized upon these educational innovations, and Harvard Medical School became identified in the public eye as a leading innovative institution, concerned with "how to make a better (and more caring, humanistic) doctor." In response, faculty who opposed tutorials and student-directed learning caricatured the New Pathway as "soft," "touchy-feely," and lacking in the intellectual rigor of the "hard" sciences. "Basic scientists" went on the attack and succeeded in reducing the curricular hours devoted to the behavioral sciences, eliminating a quite successful new course on the human life cycle. The fundamental question that emerged throughout these debates was whether students educated in the New Pathway would acquire the requisite "fund of knowledge, attitudes, and skills" to make them competent clerks and ultimately, clinicians. It was in the context of these debates that the traditional curriculum was dubbed "the classic curriculum," thereby providing identification for its students and faculty with "proven" clinical competence and with the many residents and faculty physicians similarly educated whom they would encounter in clinical rotations in their third and fourth years.[2]

The most vociferous debates in the early years of curricular development and institutionalization were carried out by faculty engaged in teaching the basic sciences, in part because these changes reordered departmental power measured in terms of control over the content and teaching of preclinical courses. The innovations also progressively challenged departmental boundaries and traditional educational hierarchies as interdisciplinary courses were developed and institutionalized. Students remained attuned to faculty questioning the "competence" of the educational process, and it was not at all surprising that during the first two years of medical school, student concerns about becoming competent clinicians focused on curricular issues.

Even as revolutionary change was being institutionalized in the preclinical curriculum, supported by many clinical faculty who taught in the new basic science and patient-doctor tutorials, the conservators of clinical competence maintained dominant training authority in the hospital-based third- and fourth-year clinical clerkships. Most residents and attendings (faculty physicians) who trained students in the practice of medicine were but tangentially involved in, and at times, remarkably ignorant of, the substance of the New Pathway's preclinical innovations. Many regarded the innovations as deviations from the "classic curriculum" in which they had acquired their basic fund of knowledge. When clinical faculty and residents disparaged aspects of the new curriculum through offhand comments and casual remarks, student anxiety increased markedly. Clearly the residents and clinical faculty continued to be the primary players who defined, created, and produced "professional competence" in medical work. How does this happen?

The Anxiety of Not Knowing What to Know

Student anxiety about mastering the "fund of knowledge" considered necessary to perform in clinical clerkships mirrored faculty anxiety and peaked during the initial years of curricular innovation, particularly for the New Pathway students.[3] Although the case-based tutorials introduced through the New Pathway were viewed by many students as a far more compelling way to learn the biomedical sciences, the new curriculum was regarded as experimental and fraught with problems of the "new."

Many students, even those who would not have entertained pursuing their medical education through the classic pathway, fretted: What did they need to know? What did the evaluations mean? Why were there no quantitative tests of their knowledge, as in the classic curriculum? Would they perform well on the medical boards? Would they do as well as their classmates who had the benefit of the "proven" classic curriculum? Would they appear as competent as the classic students when they began their clinical clerkships? Would hospital attendings and medical faculty disparage their preclinical education, as had some unconnected with the innovations, not only to students but to the press and media as well? Such questions colored the preclinical years, spilling into classroom discussions.

Although few students in the classic curriculum publicly questioned the competence of *their* program and faculty, New Pathway students often fervently questioned the very "competence" of their curriculum and faculty to turn them into knowledgeable and skilled physicians.

Most students managed their anxiety well, and a few appeared strikingly self-confident from the onset of the "experiment." Others developed confidence over the course of the first two years as they assessed that what they were learning was what they needed to know. Students well educated in the basic sciences prior to medical school "cruised" through their first year, regardless of educational pathway; many found the second year of pathophysiology (or New Pathway variants) exhilarating as they learned to think like physicians about diseases and the biomedical sciences. For a few students, especially those educated in the New Pathway, confirmation that they had acquired an expected "fund of knowledge" that readied them for clinical clerkships and the care of patients came only after their second year when they passed the National Medical Board Exam (Part One).

Although students claimed they were "terrified" at the amount of information for which they were responsible, the social context that produced intense group-wide anxiety soon changed. Initial distress abated as faculty and administrators increasingly legitimated curricular changes and students entered the realm of clinical medicine. By the end of the second year, students discovered they were readily integrating basic science and clinical knowledge, "putting the pieces of the puzzle together," and "filling in the gaps" by "knowing the right questions to ask."

The Harvard students who participated in our study had variable clinical experiences prior to entering third-year clerkships. Students from the New Pathway and a small contingent of classic pathway students were involved in longitudinal courses devoted to basic clinical and interviewing skills, to analyzing the "psychosocial" and preventive aspects of clinical medicine, and to exploring dimensions of the patient-doctor relationship. Most classic pathway students participated in an intensive twelve-week introduction to clinical medicine at the conclusion of their second year. Students ranged in their misgivings about how clinically competent they would be when they entered third-year clerkships, and many claimed, albeit with humor, that the new responsibility for patients "terrified" them. The intense emotional language, often expressed without the affect, allowed students to capture the immensity of what they considered to be their next step—taking responsibility for patients also meant taking responsibility to be "clinically competent." Regardless of tales of humility and uncertainty—a ritualized self-deprecation at the end of the second year—students were "chomping at the bit" and anxious to "do what I came here to do . . . take care of patients." But what indeed did taking care of patients mean? What would clinical competence entail?

Presentation and Performance

When you get to clinical clerkships, one of the biggest problems . . . that you deal with, I think, is developing a differential diagnosis. . . . Talk about having to change your way of thinking! This, this was the big difference, now. It wasn't . . . well what is the answer? It is: what are all the possibilities? . . . There are very few disorders in which just one thing will give you . . . the answer, give you the diagnosis. You have to do some detective work. . . . It's sort of . . . creative problem solving.

—Third-year clerk, classic pathway

As medical students proceed from basic science education through clerkships in clinical training, they move from the anxiety of not knowing what to know, to the artifice of presentation and performance. "Performance" emerges as a dominant, recurring theme throughout clinical training, a metaphor about displaying evolving competence to the hierarchy of residents and faculty physicians.

Yet "performance" also means acquiring judgment and clinical reasoning and learning the narrative strategies to present "what medicine cares about" in interactions with the training audience, the attendings, and residents. And early clinical interactions quickly teach students the nuances and variability of what is regarded as medically relevant. As in the classic study of socialization in medical education, *The Student Physician* (Merton, Reader, and Kendall 1957), students continuously assess what clinical faculty care about, balancing these lessons with what they observe and learn from interviewing and examining patients. Presenting patients in requisite ways and creating clinical narratives meaningful to the clinical service eventually lead students from experiencing the artifice of "performance" to the power of narrative competence that leads to actions on behalf of patients. As students gain clinical maturity, their comprehension of performance deepens. Their concerns shift from presentations of patients for attending physicians and residents to the creation of competent clinical narratives that influence the care of patients and the outcome of treatment.

BECOMING A CLERK

Clinical clerkship rotations brought students a markedly different learning experience from the basic sciences, regardless of educational pathway. Nearly all found that "stepping onto the wards" led to "astonishingly steep learning curves," not only in cognitive forms of knowing but also in embodied skills and ease in caring for patients.[4] However, the clerkships introduced new uncertainties about how to be competent in medicine, surgery, pediatrics, obstetrics, neurology, and psychiatry; how to perform, present patients, behave, and—yes—please one's intern, resident, attending, and team.

Being "competent" in one setting did not necessarily translate, students argued, to another. "It's intern-dependent," (or attending- or service- or hospital-dependent), they exclaimed as they offered examples of capricious or arbitrary evaluations, or positive "unique" experiences that taught them special techniques, gave them responsibility, reined them in for interpersonal or behavioral transgressions, or rewarded them for being "cheerful," "good medical students." Taking care of patients and learning medicine involved a great deal of team time. Indeed, students often spent far less time interacting with patients than with their interns and residents. Yet students reported that the experience of becoming competent through the clinical rotations was highly individualized, a sharp contrast to the collegial learning and shared responsibility characteristic of the first two years of tutorials and conference seminars. Nevertheless, as students related stories of their personal quest to become competent physicians, common experiences emerged over and over again. Talk about performance and presentations dominated discussions about learning clinical competence in these early clerkships.

PRESENTATION OF SELF: "HMS SO AND SO"

Student humor highlights the daily interactions in the clinical rotations, which produce and reproduce experiences of becoming competent in different medical settings. Performance, as a core metaphor, includes not only the presentation of patients—orally on rounds and in written form—but the presentation of "self." Clinical and medical knowledge and skills, and even hard work and responsibility, necessary to "getting the job done" in caring for patients, are but part of requisite performance. Some students discover, often to their surprise, the difficulties of presentation of self; whereas others, even those who seriously worried about their mastery of knowledge in the sciences basic to medicine, discover that they excel. The variability of these experiences eventually sorts students into specialties.

Students joke—without prompting—about the ideal clerk, the Harvard Medical Student, "HMS So and So." Cheerful, enthusiastic, bubbly if on pediatrics, "sweet" if female, funny if male, they offer succor and assistance, and even flattery, to residents and interns. So imbued with performance, students readily reenacted these roles in our interviews with all the affective intonations of reading a "script."

HMS So and So would always have a clean white coat and would always be smiling and would . . . cheerfully support his interns and residents and laugh at their jokes. "I'll do that for you. Sure I'll take care of that. Do you want me to get you some dinner?". . . Then, at the same time, you're xeroxing articles and distributing them to your team on rounds saying, "We have this interesting case and here's something that might help you," and writing up excellent write-ups and so on. But a large part of it is the way that you perform for them as a kind of cheerleader, servant, psychotherapist, all those things. . . .

There are people who can perform like that because they are like that. (Male Harvard medical student)

"How are you today HMS So and So!" "Oh, life is wonderful. I am having such a great time. Urologic specialties are just what I've always wanted to do, and this is my chance, and oh my, this is all so wonderful, you are all so great!" (Female Harvard medical student)

A woman student laughingly produced a similar ebullient image, adding that "HMS So and So" is always "sweet and patient." Other students remarked on the necessity of being "fun," "enthusiastic," "interested," and never appearing "bored," "too aggressive," "diffident," "flippant," "complaining," or overtly expressing doubts about the competence and knowledge of faculty physicians, residents, and interns. In their more serious reflections, students remarked on faculty and team expectations that the fundamental behavior of all students, regardless of clinical clerkship, must be to have "a genuine sense of caring for your particular patients you were following, hard work, and basically, diligence."

Although student commitment and affability are highly valued, learning to produce "what medicine really cares about" in each of the clinical rotations draws students ever deeper into the world of medical knowledge and practice, a world in which the foundation is laid and experience built throughout the preclinical years. (See B. Good 1994: chapter 3.) The language of medical science and patient-physician relationships acquired in the first two years of training, and the medical gaze—the new way of seeing and thus constructing an entirely new biological world—become honed and deepened through the presentation of patients to the training team. These performances, central to the educational and clinical task, lead students in the work of culture of contemporary medical practice by teaching narrative strategies in the presentation of a case.

Learning Narrative Strategies in Case Presentation: What Do We Care About?

We used to joke about what they would do to us in our oral presentations. The joke was, they'd say "OK Jason, why don't you tell us about the patients, just quickly, just give us a bullet, just like you know, a couple of sentences, just a sentence, just tell us in about five words, give us one, tell us one word about this patient" [laughing]. That's what it was like. . . . You'd find yourself just trying to say as little as you possibly could, and if you didn't, they would run to the—you know they were on their way to the next bed anyway. So I very much had to learn in those two weeks [of medicine clerkship in the emergency room] what was the absolute minimum that we needed to know. What do we care about? "What do we care about?" is the hardest question in all of medicine!

Whether students begin their clerkship work in internal medicine, such as in emergency medicine as recounted in Jason's joke, in surgery, in pediatrics, or in neurology, performance is condensed in student experience in how to "present" patients. Many students recalled how embarrassed they were when they gave their first patient presentation, which included "a medical student history" with "irrelevant details," both medical and psychosocial. A typical comment follows:

My problem with presenting was that I would insert extraneous information, and that's not tolerated in the presentation because they go "okay, okay, okay," and it's so painful to see. So my style of being anal compulsive and putting in every little thing that I knew was better adapted to write-ups than to oral presentations. It wasn't until I got into my medicine clerkship that I learned how to give a quickie.

Several students were overly cryptic, misjudging and confounding time constraints with what was deemed by a team or attending to be medically or educationally relevant. Appropriate performance, assessing "what we care about," comprised more than working hard and being knowledgeable about the bioscience of disease processes. Lamenting his misjudgment, one student recalled his confusion:

Let's say you did the worst thing, which was to do something wrong and waste a lot of other people's time. . . . See, my problem was that I talked too short. . . . My goal . . . was not to waste people's time, probably more than it should have been. You have to waste some people's time to endear yourself to them.

Students soon learned they might be harshly criticized when they gave unacceptably imprecise, awkward, or overly long presentations but rewarded in small ways for concise, substantive presentations that demonstrated they were acquiring clinical reasoning. As they honed their own performances and came to be less tolerant of others for "wasting time," students learned not only how to ask the "right" questions of patients but to present the "right" answers, tailored to the clerkship and situational context. For example, emergency-room hand-offs—the passing of patients to the next shift—required bullets, very *brief* case presentations.

The following comments on learning to judge what is important in a given clinical context convey experiences of many students.

As a medical student, you are constantly trying to figure out what do they care about? What do they want to know? So that was when I learned how to do a presentation very, very speedily. . .

You'd start writing down the chief complaint as it was coming out of [the emergency-room patient's] mouth. So that was when I think I learned to scale things down.

Anxiety about presenting on surgery rounds, where brevity and precision are demanded, afflicts even those who identified with the specialty.

I was always nervous. . . . [The attending surgeon:] "What's the only thing I want to hear." . . . [Me:] "He's got bowel sounds." . . . [Surgeon:] "Perfect!"

Discovering a specialty that fit with one's terse, often unrewarded presentation style was a relief.

The presentation is nothing in surgery. . . . I'm very happy to talk for ten seconds about a patient, and the shorter the better.

Morning rounds, characterized as "lightning rounds," when presentations were brief—"thirty seconds is what it ought to be"—were challenging, even exciting. "I prided myself . . . I really worked on [brevity] because I thought it really added to the efficiency of the team and their progress, on morning rounds." Writing notes later in the day allowed for a different form of learning how to frame what medicine cares about.

At morning rounds . . . the junior resident recites the orders, the intern writes them, and the medical students just sort of stand by and try to glean any knowledge they can from what's going on. . . . Morning rounds is not a time when students can ask questions, because it's sort of lightning rounds. . . . The goal is to get finished with them as quickly as possible. . . . But later in the day, we have plenty of time to think about the patient and what was done, the orders that were written . . . and that's a good opportunity for students to try to figure out what's going on with a given patient. And when they [the students] pick up a patient they have to write a note on the patient every day.

So they become immediately acquainted with the care. (Third-year student commenting on a medicine rotation)

MEDICAL NARRATIVES VERSUS LIFE STORIES

Although clinical clerkship presentations varied by morning rounds, attending rounds, work rounds, and morbidity and mortality reviews, and oral presentations and written cases differed in structure, format, and detail, students discovered that to be considered competent medical students, they must undo the common-sense narratives of patients. Nevertheless, throughout the clinical rotations, students were encouraged to learn new narrative forms, to create medically meaningful arguments and plots with therapeutic consequences for patients. In this process, they sharpened their biomedical "gaze" and developed their clinical reasoning.[5] Throughout these exercises, the "psychosocial" aspects of most patients' illnesses, their social histories and emotional states, and their lives outside of the hospitals and clinics were largely irrelevant; these data from daily life were often regarded as "inadmissible evidence" in the presentations made during everyday work rounds. In the early months of clinical rotations, the pursuit of a differential diagnosis, the medical sleuthing, became supreme.[6] This pursuit was explained by a student who had recently completed his first clinical rotation in medicine.

When you see something, a sign or a symptom, or a lab value, the first thing that should happen, in theory at least, is that a differential diagnosis should pop into your mind. That is to say, what are the top five things that could lead to this lab value abnormality, . . . to this physical sign or symptom that this person is manifesting? In a sense, the first two years are important because they can give you that knowledge base you need to develop, to get the differential diagnosis. . . . Then you have to go through the process of an algorithm of your top five, then look for other things. It's sort of detective work, in a way. . . . That was what I really loved about medicine." (Third-year student speaking about medicine, his first clerkship)

NARRATIVE STRATEGIES, INCONCLUSIVE CASES, AND THE "HMS WRITE-UP"

Students discovered early in the clerkship rotations that "the HMS write-up" should ideally be structured as an argument. Designed to complement the oral presentations and to highlight the medical team's efforts at detective or investigative work in pursuing and analyzing differential diagnoses, write-ups often followed an open but persuasive format. Influenced perhaps by the tradition of morbidity and mortality rounds and by the clinical pathological conferences published weekly in the *New England Journal of Medicine,* the ideal case write-up allowed for inconclusiveness.

The basic format of the inconclusive written case was modeled after the paper cases of the New Pathway tutorials and the classic curriculum's case conferences during the first two years of medical school. (Students would devote a week to exploring the bioscience and possibilities of a case, rather than quickly determine the "right" answer.) It also conformed with the culture of internal medicine, which emphasizes the asking of questions in the learning of medicine and the open and inconclusive case. The argument form also shaped students' perceptions of what was medically relevant and how one creates medical findings that can be acted upon in caring for patients.

The "HMS write-up" and the medical argument were described by many students. The most impressive dissection was by a woman I frequently interviewed. She explained:

The good HMS write-up is to say "these are all the things it could be and this is why it's not any of them, and this is why I think it's this." But then what you always do, the good thing is to say, "in order to accept this we then have to follow this plan. We have to investigate this and investigate this." So *a good write-up will leave the question open, and will acknowledge, and should acknowledge, all of the ambiguity.* So it shouldn't conclude, but it's the first step in bringing towards that conclusion, what you want, because you will have a working hypothesis by the end even if you've left all this doubt. But as the days go by and the write-ups get shorter and the blurb presentations get shorter and you're waiting for test results and the curiosity dies down and you feel like you've done your investigative work, that's when you start creating this answer.

MEDICAL MYSTERIES AND
CASE CONFERENCES

How one leaves the question open and how one begins to create an answer were also modeled by morbidity and mortality conferences. A student who was given the rare opportunity to present twice at morbidity and mortality conferences during his medicine clerkship recalled the challenge to shift from the usual oral presentation appropriate for attending rounds ("the seven-minute format") to a format "completely different." Expectations for the case conference included a condensed version, "under three minutes," of "everything that was pertinent" (all test results) without giving away the final diagnosis and outcome. By modeling and observing the reaction of the chief resident to the morbidity and mortality presentations of residents, and with the help of his junior resident, the student learned how to set up a case "in such a way that there would be a logical stopping point" prior to revealing the final diagnosis. He told a story about presenting the case of a patient who suffered from a confusing series of postsurgical complications when she came under his care. After his brief introduction to the case, the chief resident opened discussion to the floor:

This was when people shout one thing and shout another, and this is what he loves, this is what he wants, this is what it's all about. It's a learning experience. You know, "What's the differential, what could this be?" [Each diagnosis was evaluated and discussed.] "A good idea," "a possibility," "not likely," "not a bad idea." And then he asked me to finish. So I stepped back in and then actually told everyone what happened. And boy—was there a huge gasp when I told them [a congenital hole in the patient's heart caused an atypical tricuspid valve prolapse]. . . . This is the kind of thing that hasn't been seen in years!

Such conferences build students' analytic abilities and develop clinical reasoning. They also teach the narrative strategies that frame responses to the question, *What does medicine care about?*

Building mystery into a clinical story with the intent to enhance learning leads to appreciation of "fascinomas."[7] The student who presented at morbidity and mortality conferences told me that he was particularly intrigued by patients whose problems he could not quickly diagnose; he would visit them daily and track them through the various surgical and medical services in which they were treated. He was particularly attentive to the lady with the atypical tricuspid valve prolapse:

As my intern told me, a good case is one where you don't make the diagnosis, ah . . . for an hour. A great case is one where you don't make the diagnosis for a day. But if it takes a week to make the diagnosis, now that's what they call, a fascinoma . . . and this lady was clearly a fascinoma.

Students reacted in different ways to the search for and appreciation of "zebras" and fascinomas. Some found that good care for patients with ordinary diseases at times suffered in the quest for the unusual and interesting case. "When a medical student hears hoof beats outside the window they think horses; when the attending hears hoof beats, they think zebras." Yet most students appreciated the clinical puzzles that intrigued their senior residents and attendings.

Complex Narratives and Therapeutic Consequences

Creating complex clinical narratives occurs more frequently as students gain confidence in their clinical reasoning and in their own abilities to judge and shape the more existential meanings of what medicine cares about. Students progress from simply and concisely presenting patients in a format standard to specific specialties and clinical services to fashioning clinical data with larger purposes than conveying information or pleasing the team hierarchy through performance or efficiency. The ability to craft complex narratives that have multiple purposes is a leap in narrative strategy and style, a development from the simple to the complex. This leap into a new narrative strategy emerges during the course of third- and fourth-year clinical rotations. When I compared interviews from early in the third year of training with those from later in the third year and the fourth year, students no longer spoke about appropriate formats, performances, and evaluations. Instead we talked about the nuances of crafting write-ups and presentations to persuade or to effect desired action in patient care and discussed the appropriate and inappropriate use of chart notes.

By year four, many students regularly engaged in crafting "medical mysteries" and "medical persuasion" stories in chart notes and presentations. These two genres of clinical narratives required some risk-taking as students found themselves confronting the training hierarchy or manipulating attendings to encourage alternative treatments they or their interns considered more appropriate for particular patients.

Sleuthing and crafting medical mysteries became professional play for students who were gaining confidence in their own clinical efficacy. After recounting how she and her roommate would read each other "the plot" of the weekly *New England Journal* case presentations (clinical pathology conferences) to see how quickly they "could get it" (the diagnosis), yet questioning if clinical pathology conferences are "really sophisticated" or simply "institutionally weird," one student told of "sleuthing and crafting" a medical mystery. Throughout her story, she reflected on how she felt compelled to frame her case notes and suggestions to the attending and residents on her team

in such a way that would allow her to shape the case and yet acknowledge her status "as medical student at the bottom of the hierarchy."
She relished this work.

I [acquired] this case in neurology . . . [a man who] had already been in the
hospital for . . . three weeks . . . who had come in with dementia. [But] he'd
been an accountant before, completely in charge of his own and his family af-
fairs, completely with it. So he had come in with dementia and a sudden onset
of bizarre headaches, really bad headaches, and a change in his gait. . . . He
got this whole workup for everything, everything, everything! Everybody was
saying "Oh, it's Alzheimer's." I didn't know that much about Alzheimer's but
I never thought it came on *that quickly*! They were looking for viruses, and
for this, that, and the other thing, and he had this head-to-toe workup because he also had anemia and he'd been losing weight. [The team is] saying,
"Well, there must be a cancer here somewhere." So he had a cancer workup
in addition. The only thing that had been significantly positive was on a chest
C-T [scan]. Looking for lung cancer, they found a little node in his medi-
astinum. They had biopsied it and it came back as non-caseating granulomas
which essentially means sarcoidosis. Everybody else said, "Oh, it's a red her-
ring." But I went to Harrison's [the standard internal medicine reference]
and read up about sarcoidosis and sure enough there is *neural sarcoidosis*—
but it usually presents with cranial nerve findings, where you get disjointed
eye-muscle coordination; those are the most common things. But there had
been a case reported in Minnesota of somebody presenting essentially like
this. So I copied the article and said to the attending, "I think it might be
neurosarcoidosis."

The attending encouraged the student to conduct a further computer
literature search, and she recorded her findings and proposed the diagnosis in the patient's chart. Two weeks later the attending ordered
a brain biopsy, and "the findings were neurosarcoidosis with non-
caseating granulomas everywhere, probably very rare although maybe
more common than people really think."

The case was remarkable and scheduled as a clinical pathology conference. The student recalled that at the conference the case was presented with the positive lymph node biopsy, and with the mystery
question, What is the [telling] diagnostic test? Several medical students
and attendings came close but missed the "answer." The presenting
neurologist then concluded the case with a few words. The student
continued her story:

And he said, "After all this work up and everything, the findings on the brain
biopsy were a complete surprise to us." I am sitting there in the back row going—"What do you mean, did this guy never read my notes or what?" You have
to be a medical student and couch it, "Well, this is one of the possibilities." I

was so bold as to write down the reference for everybody—"And here's the reference of neurosarcoidosis presenting in this manner"—but I did not say "*The diagnosis is* . . . !" I had told the attending and had made a bet with my resident for five dollars or pizza that this was going to be neurosarcoidosis. But of course it is so weird; the guy was much more likely to have AIDS or something. But it was there. I couldn't believe it.

The medical student was a bit confounded by the style in which the attending presented the case. She mused as to whether the attending was deliberately upping the suspense as he crafted the team's medical mystery:

I didn't know if this attending was playing the game or whether he . . . really never listened to me. . . . But it was really amusing. I thought of all this gaming that goes on at this hospital, all the little white-haired old men sit in the front row and ask bizarre questions. I mean, *it is kind of fun,* especially if you go and sit in the audience and you listen to this story and see if you think fast enough. But I don't know, such a funny thing!

Lessons learned underscore the intellectual puzzles and play of many case conferences; in this student's experience, lessons about hierarchy and staged performance were also vividly conveyed.

As students begin to engage in narratives of persuasion that aim to influence therapeutic decisions, especially when decisions are not obvious, they jump to a new level of clinical competence. A medical student recounted the construction of a persuasive "medical mystery" that brought desired therapeutic activity. Being successful in crafting persuasive clinical narratives confirms medical judgment and increases experiences of professional power.

One of the residents used to say, "If you want something done, if you believe a certain thing about a patient, you go to the attending that you know you can swing to your point of view." [For example] there was an elderly lady . . . you really don't think she should be operated on. You go to the cath jock who you think is most likely to have that point of view . . . as opposed to the person who says "We should send her to surgery anyway." You take it to the specific attending you think will be closest to that management of that patient.

[Question: And you present it in a story fashion?]

Right, you present it in a story fashion . . . so that the attending will come to the conclusion that you've already reached, that you want them to reach, which I think is such a scream. You don't just present the facts and let [them] make up their own mind. You present it in a *way,* and you have to do this in medicine because you can't tell everybody everything. You can't tell them every mitigating detail.

[Question: So this is a kind of shaping; why can't you tell them every detail?]

Time. People would never listen to you; people don't have attention spans that long. . . . You always tailor everything.

Tailoring presentations for context, audience, and purpose become routine narrative strategies as students transcend the script of the "ideal" medical student. As students embody clinical competencies, they shed the stereotyped performances and presentations (the HMS Write-Up, HMS So and So) of early clinical training. They also no longer experience such performances as staged and managed, the artifice oriented primarily to clerkship faculty and residents. It is at this point when students begin to risk arguing for a particular approach to patient care. As students contribute to defining *what medicine cares about,* professional competence becomes enhanced.

A Concluding Note on Educational Innovation

As medical students from the class of 1990 progressed through their clinical training, discussions of differences between the New Pathway and the classic curriculum largely disappeared. Many of the most contentious debates about the relative merits of the two curricula—about active and passive learning, problem-based versus lecture-based teaching, or hard and soft sciences—were minimally relevant to the clinical context in which "real competence" was being acquired. As students from both pathways joined together in the clinical clerkships, they were similarly trained and judged for competence in performance by the training faculty. Over time, as students began to have standing in the clinical hierarchy, their competence came to be linked with responsibility for patient care. As competence became embodied in student experience and in increasing abilities to craft subtle narratives that influenced patient care, debates from the preclinical years appeared ever less relevant.

Nevertheless, differences between the two curricula appeared to have some lasting effect on specific analytic competencies. The patient-doctor curriculum systematically taught the early New Pathway cohorts how to recognize, assess, and treat the psychosocial problems of patients, and New Pathway students exhibited greater skills than the classic pathway students in this domain (Block and Moore 1994; Moore, Block, and Mitchell forthcoming). In addition, the emphasis on self-directed, case-based learning fit well with current trends in medical science and medical practice encountered in the teaching hospitals (see Adelstein and Carver 1994 for additional essays on the New Pathway). However, given that the clinical faculty and residents are largely responsible for producing and reproducing clinical competence, innovations in these processes and in the meanings of competence they define will have to focus anew on clinical training settings and on those speaking and writing practices that have seldom been the object of curricular change.

CHAPTER SEVEN

The Social Production of Physician Competence

- *. . . . a hideous, terrible experience.*
- *I loved being there. It was fun, it was great.*
- *Awful, an unqualified and awful two months. Bizarre.*
- *I felt like an intern and my evaluation said I performed like an intern.*
- *I'm a pediatrics kind of guy.*
- *I'm not aggressive enough to be with all those surgeons.*
- *These times are so packed with interaction, and things are embedding themselves in your mind for you to remember.*
- *You'll remember whether you know it or not. . . . It's shocking and it's unexpected and . . . visceral . . . engaging and . . . [it gave] an edge of urgency to what I was doing.*

(Third-year students reflecting on clerkship experiences)

"Working hard and knowing a lot are not enough to get you honors!" Students were surprised when these personal qualities they claimed for themselves did not automatically lead to the sensibility that one was a competent medical student and would in due course become a competent physician. Over and over again in interviews and conversations, students remarked that they discovered that competence in medicine is a socially produced sensibility; it develops and is shaped through interactions with attendings, residents, and interns throughout the course of clinical clerkships.[1] Students frequently told stories

143

about the importance of these interactions, and how their own sense of competence could be enhanced in a given clerkship or surprisingly and dismayingly diminished. Although by the conclusion of the second year students are well aware that interactions with faculty and residents in the training hierarchy will determine the quality of their clinical experiences and the kind of knowledge and skills they will acquire during a clerkship rotation, their realization of the extent to which their performances and the faculty's evaluations are socially created deepens significantly throughout their clinical rotations. This deepening appreciation—a highly attuned sensitivity—colors how students assess a particular rotation, how they perceive and interpret their evaluations by residents and attendings, and how they regard their future options for residency training.

Throughout the clerkship years, students develop a heightened attention not only to official evaluations but to the daily backstage actions of unofficial and informal judgments, and thus students become initiated into the professional discourse on physician competence. Sensitivity and a hyperattention to the largely informal evaluative discourse often occur during emotionally laden and at times dramatic learning contexts, as students experience exhilaration at assuming responsibility for patient care, are shamed in public for "being stupid" or feel personal regret at "not knowing," and become angry and confused at what they regard as abusive or unfair judgments by their seniors of their "fund of knowledge," abilities, or potential. The sensitivity to informal and formal evaluation is taught through apparently simple daily interactions in the clinical clerkships, and for most students it becomes internalized, to be carried throughout their professional lives. Competence thus becomes a fundamental symbol in the practice and politics of American medicine, in large measure because of the daily interactions and practices in early training experiences in which intense affect is associated with evaluative discourse.

There is a remarkable similarity in the affective content of many of our interviews with medical students and with practicing physicians. As physicians and medical students come to depend upon informal as well as formal evaluative actions of professional colleagues, faculty, and peers when they assess their own medical competence, sensitivity to interactions with colleagues can lead to intense self-scrutiny as well as to comparisons to and competition with others throughout the training and medical hierarchy. In some cases, sensitivity to these evaluative interactions may also lead to an avoidance of other physicians.[2] Such early experiences in training come to color professional life and give force to the intraprofessional discourse on medical competence.

Individually defined and internalized meanings of competence evolve during these years of clinical training as well, and the quest for competence is often marked by key struggles with moral content and personal consequences. These struggles in particular provide the elementary and fundamental bases for the reflective discourse on competence in which physicians and medical students frequently engage. Performance continues to be a central organizing theme. Students reminded me throughout our interviews that how one performs and how one is judged are contextually shaped, varying by training context and clinical teams in an often disconcerting way.

I close this chapter with a proposition that by the conclusion of the fourth year, students have learned a repertoire of ways to speak about and evaluate their own competence as well as that of their colleagues and seniors. Some are well on their way to developing a "professional moral voice" in which to express disagreements over patient care and to discuss treatment errors. Seeking a professional niche in which their abilities and professionally crafted selves are valued, students often choose residencies with an eye to what specialty would most enhance their sense of professional competence.

Variability in Experience

Two disparate experiences strike students as typical of their clinical training in third-year clerkships. Clinical skills and knowledge increase "a hundredfold" (as many students remarked, often thrilled with their transformation), progressively becoming embodied and "second nature." Most students rapidly learn to hone case write-ups, chart notes, and presentations of patients to what is considered medically significant in given clinical contexts. Yet, despite an exponential increase in clinical and analytic abilities, the *experience* of becoming and being competent varies from rotation to rotation in nonlinear, substantial, and at times frightening ways. Some students emerge from third-year clerkships with a raft of excellent evaluations and few scars inflicted by training experiences. However, most found that not all of the medical and surgical specialties offered them a niche in which they and their abilities would be valued; even an elementary sense of competence was not always easily achieved.

What makes the experience of becoming clinically competent so erratic and diverse, by student and by rotation? How does it come to be perceived and reported by students as not particularly dependent on one's fund of knowledge but rather dependent on interactions with a particular training team? How do residents, attendings, and interns exert such extraordinary influence over students' sense of self-efficacy and over clinical learning and interest? Formal evaluations at the conclusion of each clinical rotation, to which residents as well as attendings contribute, are but a minor part of this puzzle of power and influence.[3]

Reflections on the importance of interactions were commonly recounted; they bubbled to the surface of our discussions without deliberate prompting and regardless of students' overall clinical experiences. About to graduate, a fourth-year student looked back on his clerkship years:

Let me just say about competence, that sense of competency, it's not a linear progression in any sense. It's so much contingent upon the people that you're working with and how they use you and how they work with you. . . . It's not something that grows, and it's very specific to the rotation that you're doing at the time. There is this sense you are mastering basic things [and that increases over the course of the third and fourth year] . . . but a lot of what made me feel so competent in March [in pediatrics] was also that I was working with people who respected me and treated me right and fairly. And I was very motivated to do the work and to learn about my patients, so that I did all the extra stuff. I took it very seriously. I identified so with the interns that I wanted to live up to their standard and I did. The following month [in surgery] I was so alienated from everybody that I couldn't even make the attempt. If they had allowed me the opportunity, I couldn't have because I wouldn't.

A third-year student accepted the variability of judgment as the norm: "This is extraordinarily dependent on who your interns and residents and even attending physicians are, because it is highly variable, even in the same hospital, ah, to what is valued in a student."

TRANSCENDING THE TRAINING HIERARCHY

Subtle transgressions of assumed traditional training hierarchies in which the medical student "is at the bottom of the totem pole" create opportunities for students to transcend the training hierarchy, to identify with those in senior positions who are more skilled, more "competent." Such opportunities enhance students' sense of competence but are often created by attendings and residents with educational intent and by interns because of the need for assistance. Experiences, even fleeting ones, when the traditional hierarchy is transcended and the assumption of patient care and apparent responsibility are "mixed up" empower students, giving them a sense of their own efficacy and abilities.

The range and variety of transcendent actions highlight how students perceive their own generative and creative role in "mixing up" the hierarchy. Being serious and motivated, taking opportunities to "bond" and identify with one's seniors (residents, interns, and attendings) and to immerse oneself in their activities, produces intense clinical learning. For all students' humor and jokes about "HMS So and So," enthusiasm and upbeat, aggressive engagement often produce experiences that transcend the hierarchy. Attending physicians craft these experiences in a variety of ways; creating apprenticeship activities that express faith in a student's ability to learn rapidly and to contribute to the efforts of the team are among the most successful teaching techniques. One student enthusiastically described this approach.

I loved OB, absolutely loved it. Part of what I loved about it was that it was very easy for me to make relationships with the staff, and I had the most wonderful time. I loved delivering babies, . . . working with the midwives, . . . arguing about how to practice OB . . . so I felt like this was a field in which I could argue and debate with people . . . so that was great! . . . The faculty were wonderful. . . . I met several physicians that I would consider my heroes. . . . It was a clerkship that worked very well for being very independent . . . and I got to first assist everybody (in gynecological surgery), and I was really needed, instead of it being the attending, the resident, the intern, and the medical student. (Third-year clerk, spring)

Taught by attendings she considered "competent, precise surgeons, really caring people," the student was thrilled by her experiences on the obstetrics/gynecology rotation. Teaching entailed not simply being *lectured to* ("they let me argue and debate"), but being *apprenticed to* attendings who led her through a variety of surgical procedures. One attending, to whom the student attached herself, had the faith to "let me do a D and C completely by myself" and walked the student step by step through the procedure. Other attendings were equally available, to teach procedures such as tubal ligations—"I did the second half"—to "sewing" on Caesareans. The student was fortunate to be treated by her obstetrics/gynecology attendings as "part of what goes on" and expected to contribute in a valuable way. They assumed she might bring more recent medical knowledge and appreciated her assessment and understandings about patients. The traditional and expected training hierarchy with the medical student at the bottom was transcended, and thus learning through practice was intensified.

Negative experiences, when students are discounted and their contributions considered unimportant, reinforce the expected hierarchy and instill frustration and a sense of disesteem. The following vignette—a negative experience with an intern in pediatrics—illustrates how students are attuned to subtle interactions that convey their value or lack thereof even to those next lowest on the totem pole, the interns.

I would spend the entire afternoon . . . calling about labs and things, and then I'd go to the intern: "These are the lab results for the day, this is what I think we should do" . . . or "This culture came back positive for this" . . . and they'd go, "Oh, I knew about that hours ago, the lab called me, I already wrote for the antibiotics," which is like "Thank you very much!"

The interpretation that students had little to offer in the daily tasks of caring for patients was often triggered by the dismissive actions or surly behavior of interns.

WORKING AT THE INTERN LEVEL

"Working at the level of an intern" in contrast to being disregarded by interns can feed a growing sense of confidence that allows students to excel. Throughout interviews and discussions, students highlighted when they had "worked at the intern level," lived up to "intern standards," and not only knew as much medicine as the interns—"it varies by the time of year"—but transcended their student role in terms of responsibility they assumed for patient care.

A story from "a pediatrics kind of guy" exemplifies how the nuances of performance "as one of them" encourage students to bond, identifying with the team of interns and residents.

That was the most wonderful month of my clinical years. It was just great. . . . I had wonderful attendings, interns. They were a great team. Suddenly, all this quirkiness of myself was allowed and . . . celebrated. I carried my tools . . . in this Pink Panther lunch box and wore choo-choo train cuff links and . . . I had the greatest time. I felt so at home and accepted. . . . I really got to learning about the patients and being on top of the patients. I knew all the intern's patients because I did cross-over stuff. I felt like an intern, and my evaluation said I performed like an intern. And it was a great experience to feel like I knew what I was doing and to feel like I really liked the people I was working with.

And later in an advanced clerkship in adolescent medicine the student experienced how an attending's expectations and trust influenced his performance and that of fellow medical students: "Dr. [M.] oversaw you with benign neglect. He sort of trusted us. . . . You really felt maybe you had earned his trust, maybe you hadn't, but you were going to live up to it." When attendings conveyed their trust in students' abilities, they encouraged students to push the bounds of their competence. The boundary between what students were expected to know and be able to do and what they sought to do in patient care was highly fluid; some students were exhilarated by the opportunities to work at the edge of their abilities. Few expressed concern that they were placed in untenable situations where they could not call for assistance and monitoring when uncertain. The balance between a watchful apprenticeship that closely monitors and teaches students and clinical situations when students are extended internlike responsibilities shifts during subinternships or advanced clinical rotations offered in the fourth year.

Learning at the Boundaries of Competence

Living up to faculty expectations—when students are pushed to the edge of their competence and stretched the boundaries of responsibility—made for many of the most exciting and compelling moments in clinical rotations. A fourth-year student recalled critical incidents from his general surgery rotation and surgical subinternship. His stories illustrate how unintended opportunities allow students to transcend the traditional hierarchy of responsibility, enhancing their experience of competence in extraordinary and occasionally disturbing ways.

The hierarchy of responsibility is fragile when busy medical services are short of residents.

The first night I was on call [in surgery rotation], the intern left at six o'clock, and I didn't realize that she hadn't written any notes on any of the patients. . . . There were twenty-five patients and I didn't know any of them so I had to stay up all night writing notes for all these patients. I had to pick up a lot of the slack on the service, but it worked out well for me in the sense that I was noticed, that I was doing this work. . . . They liked me a lot.

As the student continued to fill in for the intern (who was not performing as expected for unknown reasons), the chief resident commented to the student, "It's a bad business when you've got other people doing your work for you, real bad business." Yet for this budding surgeon, the opportunity to work at the boundaries of his competence was exhilarating. And his desire to take up the intern's work was interpreted positively by his residents, who saw him as "wanting to do the best job I could do."

What he should seek to do in caring for patients, what he was capable of doing, and what he was allowed to do were seldom clear in the advanced clinical rotations.

It was always the hardest part for me, knowing where all my lines were . . . what line to draw. I didn't want to go too far and take too much responsibility but at the same time, I wanted to do everything I could do. . . . That was my biggest problem . . . but I would always try to do everything that I knew for sure I could do. Then I would sort of have to sit there and debate, "Well, can I go ahead and take out this patient's staples?" or whatever. . . . If you make a mistake and do the wrong thing, then if something happens, everybody's coming down on you. You're sort of exposed.

[Question: How is the message given or not given, what that line is?]

Most people won't explicitly give it to you. . . . There are some fine lines. . . . They size you up and say, What can this person handle? How much do they know? Then they give you as much leeway. . . . Once you become more comfortable with the person you're working for, you can take more and more leeway, and if you overstepped your bounds a little bit, they'll probably be nice and say, "Naw, I don't think you better do that because we might get in trouble."

The possibilities of taking leeway were most likely when training was secondary and covering the service became a primary reason for allowing students to work at the edge of "what they could do."

I wanted to work at the edge of what I could do. . . . I did thoracic for a couple of weeks. . . . The chief thoracic resident came down with [a debilitating disease]. . . . They were left in a bind, short a person. I'd done two weeks, was going to do another month as a subintern in general surgery. . . . They asked me to stay on the thoracic service and help them out, sort of acting as a resident. But I didn't know what my role was going to be. . . . And I loved working with the new chief resident, . . . a great surgeon, . . . a really good role model. [They] respond to me and like me and believe that I can do a good job.

They were pushing the bounds of my competence, . . . probably overstepping the bounds of my competence. They had me . . . it was really never defined what I was doing, but basically I was taking call by myself. [Because the service was short a resident there was a gap in the caring hierarchy.] I was sort of responsible for all these forty patients and ten patients in the ICU . . . so that was sort of pushing the bounds of my competence. . . . It was thrilling and I was sort of scared to death. The first night I was on call I finished all my work by one in the morning and I could have slept for four hours, but I couldn't sleep because I was too nervous. I didn't want something to happen while it was my watch. So I just ran around and checked all the patients.

Diligence, knowledge, and skills allowed the student to "sort of" become responsible for patient care. His additional weeks on the thoracic service also taught him that diligence was not the only requirements for providing good care; he also encountered the momentary limits of his "fund of knowledge" and clinical experience. He told me what he called a "hairy situation" story—a lesson to learn from and be remembered. In this particular situation, the physiological dynamics of a patient were the source of the lesson for both the student and his chief resident.[4]

A Hairy Situation. While "acting as a resident" as part of the surgical team, the surgeon-to-be became embroiled in a "hairy situation." He had been caring for a patient who had recently undergone a thoracic procedure and who was "a really sharp guy, that's how normally he was, and really had been a very, a great patient." His patient began to act "really wacked out, really acting bizarre. . . . He was old, he was about seventy years old and lots of times that happens to old people in the hospital. But I learned a great lesson from that because we saw him for a day and half." The patient became increasingly confused; the residents and surgical team believed he had high carbon dioxide levels because he had been a heavy smoker. The student felt increasingly uncomfortable as his formerly "great patient" was placed in restraints; the patient's unusual behavior was attributed to intensive-care-unit psychosis.

I guess I never felt comfortable, *but I was not experienced enough to recognize . . . The chief resident didn't recognize either what was happening.* I was on call, so I said, "Well I'm concerned about this guy, all this stuff's happened. I'm going to come by and see him."

Concern mounted throughout the evening as the patient became more and more "bizarre." His behavior and emotional state were confounding.

I was drawing blood gases during the night and his CO_2 started slowly creeping up. It was sixty-two, then sixty-three, . . . then . . . sixty-five. His status was the same. His blood pressure and everything was stable. He was fine. I don't know, *if I had been an experienced person, if I had known what was going on,* I would have stopped it about five hours earlier and said this is ridiculous, we need to check into this more. Something's wrong here. I knew something was wrong, but I waited, it was like one o'clock in the morning. I waited five hours longer than I should have. Then I said this is ridiculous. I took another blood gas. It was sixty-eight. Then I realized, something clicked, and I said, this is wrong, this is probably what's causing it. I am concerned he is getting worse.

The student called the chief resident; they sent the patient to the intensive care unit, where he was intubated "by the anesthesia people who confirmed my assessment," but "this was definitely getting beyond my abilities."

What we determined, *we all learned something,* even the attending did. First we looked back and his CO_2 when he came into the hospital was forty. It was normal. So he was not a chronic lung patient. . . . *I've been teaching this* since it happened to us . . . when you get a terrible metabolic alkalosis this is what can happen. [He described the biochemistry and physiology of the imbalance.]

Although the patient slowly recovered, the student regretted that the seriousness of the crisis had escalated: "The whole thing was much more of a flog after five hours." He mused: "If we could have identified the problem a day earlier too, we should have probably . . . *that probably was not my responsibility. No, that was the chief's, and he felt bad too. He made a mistake and so we both learned.*"

The hairy situation story cautions how being "sort of" responsible can increase patient suffering. For this student, the error committed and the lesson learned could best be rectified by teaching about a hitherto unrecognized (or ill-attended) physiological dynamic: "Few people in medicine know this, because I've been teaching it since this happened to us." Teaching as a clinical corrective indicates a significant leap in clinical maturity and competence. The explanation of error, however, centered on not only the dynamic of physiological changes and unusual physiologic causes behind the crisis but the uncertainty of who had responsibility for the patient's suffering. Thus, the student also worked through the implications of his failure, in fact his inability to identify the patient's problem more quickly, in terms of shared responsibility with those senior to him on his team. Pressed to the boundaries of his knowledge and ability to judge when a patient in crisis required intervention, the student noted not only his limits of knowledge but also those of other residents and his chief resident, who held ultimate responsibility. Yet, as the student recounted the story, he kept shifting the focus of responsibility and blame, accepting it ("if I had been an experienced person, if I had known what was going on, I would have stopped it about five hours earlier") and not accepting it ("the chief resident didn't recognize [it] either" . . . "it was probably not my responsibility").

Although the lesson learned was one of paramount importance to the student's advancement in both knowledge and responsibility during his subinternship, the lesson itself was shared. And the lesson underscored the complexities of shared responsibility for patients in surgical work and the pitfalls and benefits of such sharing. It was also a lesson in how working at "the edge of one's competence" can not only be exhilarating, creating tremendous opportunities for learning, but also entail a certain amount of risk taking and riskiness for patients in one's care. Curiously, one point buried in this "hairy situation" story—always review the chart!—was not explicitly made a part of the lesson as it was recreated and conveyed during our interview.

Enforcing/Reinforcing Hierarchy

You don't really know how well you are doing ever. It is all dependent on their feedback. And it's not just the formal feedback "oh you're doing a good job" but "we think you can take on this extra case" or . . . just the way they listen to you on rounds. I mean either they don't look at you or they look at you. That's an important message. If they look at you, you feel like you are talking to them, you feel like you're participating on their level as a colleague. If they don't listen, then you know exactly what that means—you are a student and you are being tolerated and you feel like an idiot. That's all you have to go on, there are no hard measures.

(Third-year clerk)

While transcending the hierarchy produced competence-enhancing opportunities and steep learning curves for many students, rigidly enforcing the hierarchy in such a way as to make students feel merely tolerated or disparaged created barriers to apprenticeship, interfered with bonding, and assaulted students' self-efficacy. Faculty

designed some barriers to competency and collegiality as ways of sort-
ing the type of student sought for particular specialties. Others were
clearly unintended responses, consequences of intern fatigue or attending and resident "quirkiness." Two situations illustrate common difficulties even high-performing students encountered when they failed to
fashion their behavior, and thus their "performance," to expectations
of the training team.

A student who had intended from the onset of her medical education to enter neurology earned numerous excellents and near excellents in her clerkships but found her surgery rotation trying and distressing, in part because of the way hierarchy was enforced through
the "requisite flattery" of residents—"you should elicit this little gem
that you think they know." She attributed her difficulties to divergent
expectations about performance; she and the surgical team were in serious disagreement. Although not aggressively enthusiastic about learning the surgeons' craft, she entered the clerkship not wanting to be
humiliated in the operating room. Although motivated to learn whatever she needed to know to avoid disparaging or hostile responses, she
soon discovered that

I didn't fit in with those surgeons, I was much too shy, I'm not nearly aggressive enough. . . . You can't be diffident, absolutely not. I felt the burden of
not being an ideal medical student in just how friendly people were towards
me. Feeling basically ignored, out of surgery, [on the wards] completely ignored, particularly by the chief resident. Just as if I wasn't there, at times he
would not even greet me. I felt that was definitely punishment because "if
you don't flatter me, because you don't act like a little dog—yip, yip, yip—I
am not going to speak to you because the only way our relationship is going
to work is you flattering me." It was tense.

She resisted what she surmised was expected of medical students, and
the ostracism continued. Not being engaged by the teaching staff,
marginally civil treatment, ostracism, and deliberate lack of attention
were common to student experience. These informal evaluative interactions are remembered as humiliating, painful challenges to one's
potential to become competent.

Disconfirming the abilities of students and dismissing their contributions to the tasks of a unit, ignoring questions about the mundane
workings and expectations of a service, and refusing to teach by example difficult procedures, which if done poorly are painful for patients
(such as spinal taps), contrast with the apprenticeship style of training.

Such treatment made students feel "incompetent," regardless of their accomplishments in previous rotations; the progress many students felt they had made on other clerkships was threatened when negative teaching occurred. Although varying by rotation and student (no single clerkship was commonly held as negative or destructive), these negative experiences produced a commonly held cynicism about the profession, in which "abilities" and "knowledge" were regarded at times as quite secondary in importance to "affability" and enthusiastic, managed behavior appropriate to one's position in the medical hierarchy.

Some students felt that the need to manage interactions with the training team could be regarded as an assault on personal authenticity, distorting "real" or essential competence. A fourth-year student, reflecting on negative experiences in clinical rotations, felt his knowledge and hard work were less important to how he was evaluated than his reserved, quiet style. He ruefully acknowledged his inability to overtly express "enthusiasm," and wistfully remarked that he would have preferred more observation and monitoring by faculty attendings. He believed his performance with patients and his clinical acumen and skills were far more developed than his "affability." Recalling his pediatric subinternship, he said,

If you don't make baby noises with the doctors then you—I mean I am perfectly willing to make baby noises at the baby, but I'm not going to do it with the doctors.
[Question: Is it necessary even in subinternships?]
I guess you do because once again my evaluation was, one of my favorites: "HMS X did an excellent job, . . . had an excellent fund of knowledge, got along with the patients excellently, was able to come up with excellent differential diagnoses, did excellent write-ups." Every word was excellent or outstanding. My final grade *was not* excellent.

The student explained that his resident informed him the attending who wrote the evaluation misread his reserved style for lack of interest in the specialty and in what the attending had to teach. This student proposed that "performance" had two meanings in medicine, both confounded and "muddled." Not only did one need to have the abilities and knowledge to get things done and care for patients, but "more than in most professions," medicine valued "staging and acting," and competence became "muddled" with these characteristics of "performance."

Civility and Embracing the Profession

You have to earn the right to joke around!

Embracing the medical profession entails not only the acquisition of knowledge and technique but the achievement of highly honed professional behavior that transcends the consciously managed performances of "staging and acting" during case presentations or in conferences and on rounds. Attendings, residents, and interns clearly reward students who interact with enthusiasm, diligence, and attentiveness in patient care, and who express commitment to specific clinical specialties. Interactions are also designed to curb what attendings may regard as excessive, unprofessional ebullience and aggressiveness, particularly toward the training team. Although students are frequently well rewarded with positive evaluations for exhibiting ebullience and aggressiveness, "professional civility" also becomes a training goal. Professional civility includes acknowledging one's place in the medical hierarchy and accepting a code of professional behavior in how one relates to one's peers and seniors, as well as to one's patients. For some students, the management of expressiveness with other students and physicians created more of a learning hurdle than the development of technical competence, medical judgment, and a caring manner with patients. Becoming competent in relating to and working with faculty and residents forced some students consciously to create new professional selves.

Although many students mature professionally without experiencing ontological assaults on who they essentially are, others find they must work at redefining themselves as physicians, as they seek to embrace the profession. (Some students never quite choose to embrace the profession as it is modeled at the Harvard teaching hospitals.) As one student recounted, an initial inability to "keep my mouth shut," to monitor his overengaging and ebullient behavior, "cost me honors" in several core clerkships early in the third year. As in examples noted above, the student reported that his fund of knowledge was not questioned, but his behavior was considered by some faculty as "flip" and inappropriate. His eagerness to answer questions put to other students or residents was viewed by faculty as impolitely assaulting the training hierarchy. In contrast to the ostracism experienced by some students who resisted tailoring their behavior to the particular training contexts in which they found themselves, this student felt his residents and attendings aggressively sought to draw him into the profession, deliberately but benignly reshaping his professional being. During the course of our interviews over the clerkship years, he told me about several "reining-in experiences." These experiences were personally transformative. He embraced the lessons of the profession and attained his first-choice match in a highly competitive residency program. His accounts of reining-in experiences are similar to experiences of other students who "embraced" the profession and sought to bond and identify with the training team members.

> The clerkship director sat me down and said, "You're very smart, that's apparent, but you talk too much and you've got to just sit and listen," in a nice fatherly way, not in a nasty way, kind of "you seem like a good guy, don't mess things up for yourself." So I took his advice. . . . It took three rotations, but I finally learned how, at the very least, how to play the game.

Being monitored and reviewed created discomfort but intensified his efforts at learning "to play the game."

> The sense that everything you did, I don't know if it's true or not, but everything you did was scrutinized—every little joke—"that's it, there goes my life"—was very stressful, terrible, the most stressful thing about clinical rotations.

Students often sought comfort in their fund of knowledge or technical skills when they spoke of their incompetence in interactions with clerkship team members, of criticisms of their behavior, of their failures in the "staging and acting" part of clinical performance.

> It was never that stuff [technical skills and fund of knowledge], nobody ever questioned my competence, ever. I always got pretty high marks on that. It was the behavioral things that people questioned more. . . . [Attendings would say] "You know stuff even my residents don't know but you've got to shut up." I would rather have heard comments like that than heard I'm not competent or I'm not smart because I think behavioral stuff is easier to change. I've become a very high self-monitoring person. But I was afraid that if I let them get the foot in the door, they were going to squash all the joy out of me and I would become one of the walking dead. I think I understand now that needn't be and in my peds clerkship when I was in the process of getting slammed the final day, the chief resident said something to me that really was some very good advice. "You have to earn the right to joke around."

Learning how to respond "yes sir, no sir" and "keep your white coat buttoned," exhibiting an understanding of one's sense of place in the hierarchy, can also create the experience of becoming competent in professional relationships. But such advances also create a sense of self-scrutiny, and students struggle to balance their essential selves with the demands of professional behavior.

It's a fine line, this is something I've hassled with my whole life . . . how to get someone's respect and instill confidence, yet still be funny, be human, be personable.

I am loath to set foot on a patient floor without a tie and shoes and decent clothes. . . . I've decided, given my personality and the way people perceive me, if I look very straight, that will give me a little more leeway. I've decided looking conservative is going to be my secret weapon from now on.

Small Rebellions and Developing a Moral Voice

Learning to reshape behavior does not exclude small "rebellions" directed against what are perceived as cynical or inhumane practices, especially for the majority of students who "embraced" the medical profession by the conclusion of clinical training. Minor acts of resistance are cultivated within the rules of the game and expressed within acceptable professional bounds.[5] Small rebellions vary by service and hospital, by specialty, and by colleagues and the clinical team; they may entail masking one's quirkiness in clerkships where it is not celebrated or creating circumscribed professional spaces where one's true self can emerge, one's emotions can be expressed, or one's moral commitments can be acted upon. Two stories illustrate.

Combatting the cynicism of clerkship colleagues became a goal of one student:

It's not one of the more adult coping mechanisms, classifying old patients as gomers, assuming that IV drug users are lying, assuming the worst, not having any optimism, any positive outlook. It becomes the thing to do, to make cynical comments, and it becomes a way of getting along with everyone else. . . . It's really awful. It's something I have tried very hard not to do. When I'm on a team, I often forbid the people on my team to say the word "gome" because I just hate it. It's lack of respect for the person.[6]

Highly respected by many members of her class, the student took small risks as her personal moral stance tapped into the "caring" and "humanism" of medicine, often lamented as lost by tired and cynical interns and clerks.

Admonished by an attending not to sit down when in a patient's room "because you want them to look up to you, it's not an equal relationship," another student reported he often engaged in minor rebellion, resisting the advice of his seniors.

> I think that's exactly the reason medicine's gotten into some of the trouble it [has] because doctors have set their patients up with these great expectations we couldn't meet. I've been socialized [not to sit when in a room with patients and the attending], I play the game. But when I am in the room with a patient, one on one, and there are no other docs around, *I sit down*. . . . I'm just not comfortable walking into a room looking down at a patient. . . . I'll play the game when I'm in the room on rounds with the other residents. I'll stand and I won't say a word, I won't joke around with patients, nothing, but when I'm on my own, that's something that I will not change.

These minor acts of resistance permitted students to reassert aspects of their personalities and to behave in a way they valued. These actions most often occurred as students gained confidence in their knowledge and ability to care for patients and to perform appropriately in a given clinical context. Indeed, such acts of resistance in the course of medical training not only reinforce the professional hierarchy but serve to incorporate the medical student as a young professional into the system of power and control and of individualized and professional responsibility. They also prepared students to develop a professional moral voice, the mark of a mature clinician.

Developing a Professional Moral Voice

If you feel strongly that whatever is going on isn't right, you have to find some way, as politely as possible, without sort of pointing the finger at anybody [to] say I really do think that this is a possibility and you might want to consider doing this to make sure . . .

(Fourth-year clerk, late in her senior year)

The point is to preserve the smooth social functioning in which all the bad stuff is kept out of sight. The complainer is the one who has realized what's going on and gives voice to it, but they're hated. At 7 A.M. work rounds, "Well, we have a hard day ahead of us but it will be fine." And you have this one voice of reason going "no, no, no, it's not." It's disturbing and you just want to get rid of that person.

(Fourth-year clerk)

How do students develop a professional moral voice in the face of what many physicians and social scientists refer to as "a conspiracy of silence"—when physician performance is rarely evaluated and errors are seldom spoken about in a direct and formal fashion? Although the conspiracy of silence has been pierced in recent years and an informal evaluative discourse on physician performance has flourished in many medical communities, silence regarding errors and medical mistakes is often still the norm. In medical education, the errors and mistakes of students are readily taken as examples to learn from, and expressing and modeling a moral voice is part of the task of attending faculty and residents. Morbidity and mortality conferences may lead attendings to "wear the hair shirt" in exercises of teaching, modeling, and penitence (see Bosk 1979). Clinical pathology conferences and attending conferences at times introduce new research, allowing for the redefinition of appropriate procedures, the reinterpretation of knowledge, and refinements of biomedical techniques. Silences are also modeled, however, in these contexts, and students become increasingly aware of what is not said as well as what is presented.[7]

Clerkship rotations also provide students with diverse models of how to develop and at times to silence a moral voice. Students not only learn how to address mistakes in patient care or to dissent over what constitutes the best care, but how and when to mask dissent. At times students are faced with or participate in a "conspiracy of silence," and many acknowledge the prevalence of a civil inattention to the errors or misjudgments of their seniors. Even for students who heartily embrace the profession and its codes of performance and civility, disagreements with the training team over patient care may affront their moral sensibility. Acquiring a professional moral voice and the conviction to express it remains a challenge for many students, as it does for many physicians in practice.

Moral hurdles are frequently encountered through constant and intimate interactions with residents and attendings; the behavior and performance of students are not only observed and monitored, but students in turn also survey and assess the judgment and practices of their seniors, the residents, faculty attendings, and private physicians in the teaching hospitals. Crises arise in particular when students, in their care of patients, are requested, often required, to carry out "orders" and practices with which they disagree. Situations such as those described by students often call for exceptional negotiation and a highly attuned sensibility about how to manage the training hierarchy.

Women students in particular spoke about how they learned to write notes in medical charts and to discuss cases with their residents or attendings in order to influence and affect the way in which patient care was carried out. Many recounted examples of how they would work

up a case when they disapproved of a drug regimen or procedure ordered, marshall evidence to suggest another mode of treatment, and
recommend, through a careful questioning of the ordered treatment,
a new course. The care taken in questioning a resident or attending's
practice was described in similar ways; students had to try out different approaches before learning what worked and what was acceptable,
and when and how they could rewrite an order and get it co-signed by
their residents. Most found that with residents, and even with attendings and private physicians, direct and confrontational disagreements
were seldom successful. The squeaky wheel—"no, no, no it's not all
right, and you just want to get rid of that person"—is often silenced,
sacrificed, or even "icicled" or ostracized, to maintain the smooth-
flowing workings of a team. How do students learn to voice dissent
that is not silenced?

Students caricatured conflicts with residents, fellows, and even attendings over patient care as ones which entailed the opposition of
"research" interests in esoteric diseases to the care and comfort of
patients who likely were suffering from more "mundane" illnesses. Disagreements over the therapeutic decisions frequently posed moral dilemmas for students which are conveyed in a genre of storytelling we
may call "caring for the patient." The first story recounts a critical incident from an early clinical rotation, when our storyteller was less attuned to the protocols of teaching-hospital hierarchy and less skilled
at managing residents and fellows.

I was caught a couple of times in an awkward situation where the . . . fellow—
you know someone who's already done his residency and is now specializing
and obviously knows more than the resident—would write in the chart. . . .
And I would read it and would think, "This guy knows a lot more than I do."
I'd change my order and then I would say to the resident, "Would you please
co-sign my order." And I would explain to him why I had changed it. And he
would blow up at me and he'd say, "No way, I'm not going to change it.
That fellow doesn't know blah, blah, blah." And he would assume that he
knew the right answer. And I felt real funny about it, and I felt like telling him
that he should write the order then, because I didn't want my name on something that I didn't agree with. But he practically forced me . . . so I had to
end up doing things with patients that I didn't really agree with.

Later in the clerkship the student took another tack in expressing her
disagreements and appealed to the attending faculty physician.

We had a patient with what looked like rapidly progressive Parkinson's disease. My resident was all excited about it because he didn't think it was
Parkinson's; he thought it was some new disease that he was going to

discover and put his name on. . . . In the meantime, I had taken a really careful drug history, and the guy had just gone off [one of his drugs] and his symptoms got worse after that. So I went to the attending . . .

The attending agreed that indications suggested the patient was suffering from Parkinson's and co-signed the student's order to place the patient on an appropriate drug treatment.

And so I wrote the order. And the attending co-signed it. And the next day in rounds, I said the [patient] had been started on Cynomet [a dopamine agent that would have helped symptoms of Parkinsons' disease]. And my resident blew up at me. And said, "Who wrote that order?" And I said, "Well, I did."

She told her resident the attending co-signed, that "the patient was the attending's patient," and yet was scolded for not following protocol. "No one's allowed to co-sign orders except for me," he announced to her, remarking that it was his responsibility and he would be the one called "in his sleep" if the patient suffered side effects in the middle of the night. The student felt vindicated when the attending reported that the patient

"came bounding into my office," walking normally and everything because he was responding to Cynomet. So it turned out it was the right thing to do. And I'm sure my junior resident knew it was the right drug to use . . . but he wanted to be the one to say "we should start this." This was his own little domain of power and he was going to be damned if he let anyone intrude.

As training progresses, students learn how to bring their concerns to the attention of those in power, although it is an easier task when attendings and residents are open to student contributions. Students soon discover that using chart notes to suggest other directions for treatment can be remarkably sensitive. A fourth-year student, looking back at lessons learned, told a story about a woman who had suffered a pelvic fracture at a rehabilitation hospital during physical therapy, and the student's ignorance about the sensitivity of the chart note.

I just wrote down [the patient's] story; said the patient relates this set of events [about how she felt her pelvis crack during a PT treatment]. All these people wrote notes on the chart after me . . . about how the patient doesn't remember any initiating event. . . . People cover up for each other and nobody wants to point fingers at all. Nobody wants anything in the chart that blames anybody for anything, or suggests that somebody was wrong about something.
[Question: And if errors come from outside the system?]

Usually people will just present the case in the chart as it happened and not make commentary about whether or not something was right or wrong.

She also described how she now was able to use chart notes to gain a change in diagnosis and to secure her preferred approach to patient care. Again, although chart notes were delicate tools, they could be vehicles for persuasion and even a subtle, if crafted and modest, form of dissent.

It's kind of sensitive as a student, or even as a resident, or a fellow, arguing with the attending. Especially through the chart where it's on paper. . . . You like to resolve things as much as possible through discussions on rounds. But if you feel strongly that whatever is going on isn't right, you have to find some way, as politely as possible, without sort of pointing the finger at anybody, [to] say . . . I really do think that this is a possibility and you might want to consider doing this to make sure . . .

She recounted a case during her last consultation service that concerned a patient who appeared to her to be suffering life-threatening side effects from an excessive dosage of steroids. She remarked that she had an ongoing daily discussion of the case with her attending, whom she liked but characterized rather fondly as a "lab rat." Finally, she recalled, she was able to get action on her disagreement. She based her argument on a well-researched review of the literature on the suspected "zebra" or esoteric disease and a careful review of the patient's drug history and physical symptoms. She told me how she brought the case to her attending's attention.

Well, very polite, disagreeing . . . not really arguments, but just sort of sticking to my guns, and saying, saying, "I'm not at all convinced that this isn't just steroids. I don't see any reason to think it's not." . . . This is the . . . HMS calling it a horse and the attending calling it a zebra . . . just sort of sticking to my guns and every day, in my note, politely saying "I see no reason not to think it's steroid induced."

The attending continued to argue for his point of view through the chart note as well; however, he chose to follow the treatment recommendations suggested by the student.

"Rolling your eyeballs" on rounds, "raising your eyebrows," politely posing questions phrased as "please help me educate myself about why you are doing this"—these are techniques students evolve to question choices attendings and residents make in patient care. "Gosh, that's an interesting approach to dosing that medication. Um, can you tell me how it works for you?" "Can you tell me the literature you've read that backs that up?" "Would you give a smaller dose, a bigger dose, a different medication?"—these become the repertoire of a modest, yet moral voice. Such a repertoire allows students to raise questions about the competence of those above them in the hierarchy by implying, Are you doing this for a reason? Is this just your standard, or do you want to do it this way because it is your habit?—Usually without bringing down the wrath of the hierarchy. Yet taking a moral stance requires that students have developed a sense of their own competence and the ability to judge the practices of their seniors, that they have achieved competence in exercising a professional civility. The hierarchy can also be used to advantage to change the course of patient care, but such appeals require careful preparation.

If it is something that is going to hurt the person, then you either talk to your senior resident or talk to the attending. Although again, in talking to the attending, you often have to be pretty careful not to throw blame back and forth, and people are really careful what they write in the charts. . . . Anything can happen as long as it's not written in the chart.

In our final interview, this young physician told me, in response to my question of whether there was anything that had surprised her when she reviewed the four years of medical school,

I think that I have to say one [thing] that I have never been called on to do before really and I am happy to discover that I can do . . . standing up for what I think is right in the patient's care. With lesser things I do not do it, but with things I think are important, I'll *refuse* to do something I don't think is right. Or I'll press harder to do something that I do think is right. And sometimes it doesn't work, but I've had pretty good success, and it makes me feel good about what I'm doing. And like I said, that's something I've never been asked to do before, never been in a situation where it was necessary.

[Question: Can you contrast this new sense to your previous experiences?]

It feels different now, it feels like we're all voting members. Or if I'm caring for a patient, the attending may be higher than me in the hierarchy, but we both actually have a similar vote.

Whether the gender differences I noted as I reviewed the years of interviews are evidence of a different discourse or type of storytelling by women than by men in describing their actions and "moral voices," or a manifestation of differences in the experiences of female and male students, is uncertain. Yet the women students who participated in this study often told stories of defending patients against neglectful attendings and disregarding residents, and the men told stories about how they managed negotiating power with those above them in the "ladder." A male student who talked about how he worked through disagreements with attendings over patient care acknowledged this power, as did many other male students. In response to my questions—How do you deal with disputes over patient care? Have you been in a situation where people up and down the hierarchy disagreed with the kind of care that's being given? Or with treatment decisions? How do disputes get dealt with?—he noted,

You talk about the ladder, and the ladder is based on knowledge, and so . . . if you're lower you always have to worry that the other person knows more. But I think all you really need to do is ask and they explain why. Why are we doing it this way? And for the most part, like what happens in medical services, whoever is higher up, that's the way that it's done. Because . . . other people complain about it, but it's just the way it's done and the system rolls on and people just shake their heads. The system just fluctuates really too much for there ever to be—because people are taken in and out of slots so rapidly that you never have—your seeds of discontent can never be truly sown.

[Question: And in surgery?]

Surgery is tough. You are adding another dimension; you are adding skill . . . which is only learned with time. . . . Really it's so effort dependent. . . . I hold an instrument the way, let's say, a second-year resident will, and I've been in the O.R. with interns who hold it the way an intern does. And it's a struggle, and they have yet to make that next step. You see that. There's levels of skill. But I think that the decision-making bows to the same hierarchy. I think the hierarchy may even be more strict. I think it's more strict. Because surgeons are very dependent on being fed from above.

The development of a moral voice in medicine is associated with an expanding sense of self-efficacy and competence in patient care. Formulating professionally acceptable expressions of one's moral voice, creating spaces within which one can take a personally defined moral stance or effecting action in patient care evolve as students learn how to manage the training hierarchy in their progress toward internship. Taking a moral stance and criticizing the profession from within its boundaries is also a "noble" cultural tradition, one that is not only firmly entrenched in American medicine but that is elevated to a rhetorical art by the profession's leading men and women. Perhaps in the future, the rhetorical art will also be carried forth and elaborated upon by this new generation of physicians, who increasingly will be called upon to develop clinical standards and to monitor and guide the medical competence and caring activities of themselves and their clinical colleagues.

A Valued Niche

As you begin to put your [residency] applications together, you get letters of recommendation from various people. And you get this picture of people who are supporting you and who thought well of you in your years of medical school. And it provides a little nest in which you're valued, and what you've done is good. I think for me, that separates me from all this . . . stuff that was hard to go through where I wasn't a star.

For most of us, we can be pretty good at whatever it is we are going into. We are not so much competing against each other, we are competing in a given specialty. . . . It's easy to fulfill expectations in something that you're genuinely enthusiastic about.

Students shift their concerns about competence and performance as they conclude their clinical rotations. The efforts they expend in learning to present, to perform, and to behave like ideal medical students in a variety of clinical settings are accomplishments largely internalized. By the conclusion of the fourth year, most students have acquired at minimum the basic clinical skills and knowledge expected by their faculty, and most have created a professional demeanor, some a new professional persona, with which they are comfortable. Reinforced with the knowledge that they have found a niche in the profession in which their abilities will be valued, students turn their concerns to their residency specialty and to patients they will be caring for in their internships. They describe the immensity of the change: suddenly being an "M.D." and officially declared professionally competent has consequences for patients for whom one is responsible. One is no longer primarily performing for oneself, to be judged and evaluated by one's faculty and residents. Although attention to the responses and perceptions of one's colleagues continues to be of great importance throughout residency training and into practice, there is suddenly another audience to whom one has paramount responsibility. The change, described by a new medical graduate who was soon to begin his internship, is

suddenly realizing you don't have to get yourself through the next month of a difficult clerkship, you have to get your patients through this time. . . . It's a big change. . . . Yeah, my signature counts. . . . Approaching internship I feel it very differently. I have to make sure other people get through the next month. It's a little angiogenic.

REPRODUCING PROFESSIONAL DOMINANCE
THROUGH COMPETENCE DISCOURSE

Learning competence is intertwined with reproducing the medical hierarchy and reinforcing the hegemony of professional ideologies about competence. Students take on clinical responsibilities when they have little expertise and require supervision by the training team. And they learn the repertoires of discourse professionally acceptable to challenge decisions about patient care made by those higher in the medical hierarchy when they have little status. Many students become quite skilled at these repertoires as they develop a professional moral voice in which to express concerns about patients and to engage senior physicians in practical and effective ways.

However, as the ethnographic data illustrate, students learn not only the form but the boundaries of professional critiques. They acquire not only moral but cautious voices, as they realize which repertoires are tolerated by the profession. Challenging the authority of residents or attendings against possible patient mismanagement and medical errors or standing up for patients against a possible wrong decision has to be hedged carefully to be effective and must rely on support of more powerful colleagues. Students also come to understand that medical records are public documents, and that recording disagreements or criticisms in medical charts risks breaking the boundaries of acceptable critique. In such situtations, the profession teaches that an "intraprofessional discourse on competence" should be carried out with enormous caution, often informally and out of the public eye. Thus, learning when and how to use different repertoires of discourse on professional competence reproduces professional dominance. The teaching of medical ethics from a critical perspective in which the traditional boundaries of critique are questioned may enhance the development of multiple moral voices within the profession. It may also prove rightly subversive of an unquestioned commitment to the cultural authority of the medical hierarchy.

PART III

Culture, Competence, and Clinical Science

Introduction to Part III

It's exciting, but it's a different brinkmanship. And I think for that reason you do it in a sophisticated world only, where you have checks and balances. I think these are quite separate decisions; patients may take all of that quite calmly. What they actually get out of the transaction is where they are talking and that's a separate mode and I don't think they collide really. It's a schizoid way in which you operate. One is talking to people and the other figuring out the best way to go for it. *And then telling what risks there are, and that we are very blunt about. You have to do that.*

> —Radiation oncologist, discussing experimental treatment for brain tumors

Research oncologists stand between the biosciences of their specialties and the clinical tasks of caring for people with serious and life-threatening disease that is often resistant to treatment. The "schizoid way in which you operate" identifies these two worlds of oncology—the scientific, often experimental, domain of cancer treatment and the therapeutic domain of patient care. The ability to join these two worlds in clinical work, in interactions with patients, has become one measure of specialty competence for patients, physicians, and the public. Oncologists debate how best to join these two worlds. Those who study the specialty raise questions about the tension and potential conflict of interests inherent in the two roles of the oncologist.

171

As physician-scientist, he or she must encourage patient involvement in clinical trials and experimental research protocols; as provider of care, he or she must give priority to patient well-being.[1]

In chapters 8 and 9 I explore the narrative strategies that are used by academic oncologists to join these two worlds in clinical work with patients. The previous ethnographic chapters (2 through 7) have stressed how physician competence is socially produced and given meaning through interactions among physicians, and in the case of medical education, through student interactions with the medical training hierarchy. Here I examine another facet of the puzzle of the meaning of competence and bring the patient back into the picture to address how physician competence is socially produced through interactions with patients and through the construction of clinical narratives that join clinical science with clinical care. I focus on the clinical narratives that integrate these two worlds of oncology and draw patients into therapeutic activity. It is through these narrative interactions with patients that specialty competence in clinical work and patient care (as opposed to laboratory science) is displayed, and in certain contexts, constituted.

My recent studies of the culture of American oncology and comparative analyses carried out with colleagues working in Italy, Japan, and Mexico[2] inform these interpretations. Our current study, "Clinical Narratives and the Treatment of Breast Cancer,"[3] has followed over thirty American women through their course of treatment at a major East Coast teaching hospital. Taped observations of clinical interactions and discussions with physicians about therapeutic intent, interviews with patients about their interpretations of these interactions during and after their course of treatment, and interviews with the academic oncologists who care for these patients about their clinical science constitute the research text for chapter 8. The academic oncologists are accomplished clinicians who practice on the cutting edge of advances in medical treatment, engage in laboratory or clinical research, and teach medical students and train residents.

Oncologists practicing in the United States are given a cultural mandate to instill hope by offering the latest biomedical treatments, even as they are expected to be frank in conveying the diagnosis of cancer. A generation ago, in an era of far fewer treatment possibilities, American physicians were less forthcoming in telling patients a diagnosis of cancer. Today there is virtual unanimity on the ethical and legal obligation of physicians to not only disclose cancer diagnoses to patients but to competently discuss treatment options, choices, risks, and side effects (M. Good et al. 1990; Novack et al. 1979; Oken 1961).[4] Although patients report they often encounter ambiguity when discussing prognosis, reflecting oncology's charge to maintain hope, academic oncologists in our recent studies openly discuss the uncertainties of outcome and the relative risks of primary treatments and salvage therapy (the last effort, often experimental and extremely aggressive, to reverse disease).

In American teaching hospitals and cancer centers, therapeutic options offered to patients include not only the "latest" proven anticancer treatment protocols but also "experimental" choices, thereby reflecting our society's public commitment to advancing anticancer treatments, through basic bioscience as well as clinical research. Even patient-funded cancer research for experimental treatments, an indication of our society's private commitments, flourishes. Although the ethical implications of such endeavors were briefly discussed in the mid-1980s in the medical literature (Lind 1986; Oldham 1987), the popular expectation that patients should be given choices from the cutting edge of medicine has led insurance companies to review and reconsider the costs and benefits of experimental therapies, such as bone marrow transplantation for the treatment of lymphomas, leukemias, and most recently, metastatic breast cancer.[5]

Clearly, given the inequities in health care coverage and in access to competent specialists, not all American patients receive or are offered the most effective, much less experimental, cancer care. And not all American cancer patients choose to open their bodies to "experimental" or even aggressive treatments.

The specialty practices that inform and shape clinical narratives, while tuned to the wishes of patients and to social and individual financial constraints and insurance restrictions, are deeply influenced by the broader culture and political economy of clinical and research oncology, the larger social contexts of oncology's two worlds. Although I emphasize clinical narratives and narrative strategies, I presume a model that links what happens in clinical contexts between patients and physicians with the political economy and local culture of medical practice and research. This model grew out of my comparative studies, which show that meanings of clinical competence, narrative strategies, and medical practice vary systematically across cultures and are deeply influenced by local as well as cosmopolitan cultures and political economies of medicine (M. Good et al. 1993; M. Good et al. 1994).

Specialty competence is therefore constituted not only in the context of the clinic and hospital and in interactions with patients but by the political economy of research medicine. For oncology, this includes societal investment in biomedical and anticancer research, the production and marketing of therapeutics, and the global influence of the specialty in authorizing biomedical knowledge and in defining specialty competence and standards of care. The model (see fig. 1) hypothesizes that the way in which physicians speak with patients about their diagnoses, prognoses, and treatment options (the culture of disclosure in clinical settings) is shaped by a society's ideas about medicine's role in shaping the relationship of mind and body. The culture of disclosure and of mind/body relationships thereby influences how physicians shape clinical narratives as they integrate the two worlds of clinical science and patient care. In oncology, these cultural and societal processes and the practices and institutions that produce them constitute "the political economy of hope" (M. Good 1990; M. Good et al. 1990; M. Good, Hunt, et al. 1993; M. Good, Munakata, et al. 1994). In the following chapter, I examine competence in this context of high specialty medicine.

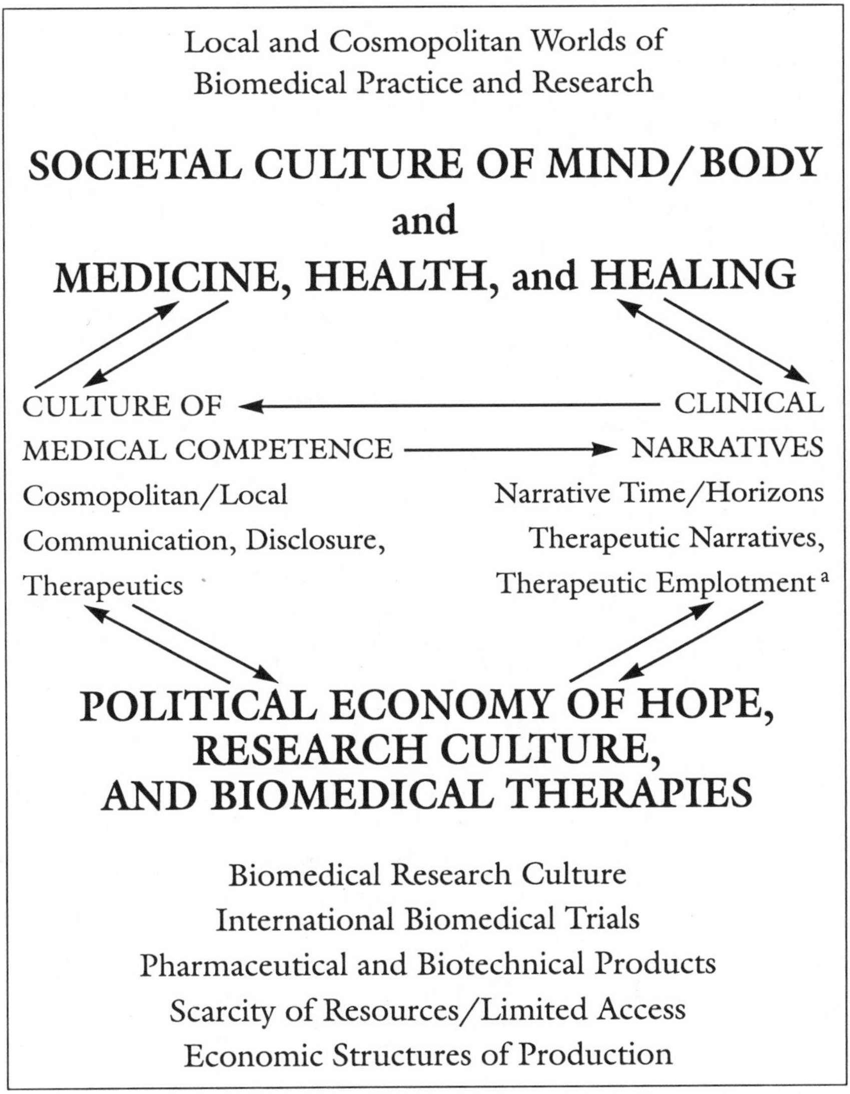

Local and Cosmopolitan Worlds of
Biomedical Practice and Research

SOCIETAL CULTURE OF MIND/BODY
and
MEDICINE, HEALTH, and HEALING

CULTURE OF ← ——————————— CLINICAL

MEDICAL COMPETENCE ————→ NARRATIVES

Cosmopolitan/Local   Narrative Time/Horizons

Communication, Disclosure,   Therapeutic Narratives,

Therapeutics ·   Therapeutic Emplotment [a]

POLITICAL ECONOMY OF HOPE,
RESEARCH CULTURE,
AND BIOMEDICAL THERAPIES

Biomedical Research Culture
International Biomedical Trials
Pharmaceutical and Biotechnical Products
Scarcity of Resources/Limited Access
Economic Structures of Production

Figure 1

[a] Cheryl Mattingly formulated the notion "therapeutic emplotment" in her research
on therapeutic narratives in occupational therapy. See Mattingly 1989, 1994.

CHAPTER EIGHT

Competence and Clinical Narratives in Oncology

Clinical Narratives

*If it's malignant, I want them to have enough informa-
tion so that they have the truth, but also so that they have
some hope. They know that there are things that can be
done that will help them. I think the hardest thing is uncertainty, and also I think it's extremely hard if you begin
to think that your doctors are not telling you things. Then
you don't know if you can ever believe them. So I find
being very frank, but not discouraging, from the beginning seems to be best. . . . Women are adults, women can
deal with breast cancer, and . . . you start out with that
assumption and you deal with them that way. . . . When
patients start out being involved from the beginning and
being in control from the beginning, it's much better. The
whole way. And treating breast cancer is a long process
these days.*

—A surgical oncologist, 1993

When literary concepts such as narrative are introduced
into observations of everyday clinical life, new aspects of medical work
and therapeutic processes become apparent. The surgical oncologist
quoted above remarked upon the importance of how she shaped the
whole story for patients, and how early clinical interactions, which she
consciously designs, give patients the experience of control over their

treatment course and ultimately over their illness. These early interactions, she contends, influence how patients cope with the lengthy process of therapy.

Oncologists have long debated how best to carry out their clinical and informational tasks with patients. Conscious consideration of how to shape patient experience has become an expected part of clinical work. How well these tasks are carried out is one dimension of an oncologist's competence in managing therapeutic activities for patients. Although contemporary clinical standards vary in patient care, oncologists invest a high degree of professional attention in this aspect of their work, as evidenced by journal articles, essays, books, and interviews. A professional discourse on the errors of physicians in carrying out these tasks appears formally in journal essays and articles, and informal judgments about clinical competence in this domain frequently emerge in research interviews with both oncologists and patients.[1]

In a complex and uncertain field like contemporary American oncology, much more than good bedside manner is at stake. Helping patients make good decisions is at the essence of competent care. Given the current state of knowledge and available therapeutics, patients must rely on the clinical judgment and skilled actions of their physicians. However, in many situations, several alternative courses of action may be appropriate. Good care includes helping patients collaborate in selecting a good course of action, but it also includes helping patients feel that a chosen course constitutes the best possible care for them. This work is accomplished through the medium of clinical narratives.

Skilled clinicians are often quite conscious of the importance of this aspect of their work, especially women oncologists who treat breast cancer patients. This awareness reflects the challenges for this specialty—to treat life-threatening disease, often over a long time, in a context of high-technology medicine but one fraught with the uncertain efficacy of therapeutic options.

NARRATIVE AS AN ANALYTIC PERSPECTIVE

Three concepts drawn from narrative analysis—plot, emplotment, and narrative time—illuminate aspects of clinical work that make clinical interactions, encounters, and information-conveying into integrated treatment narratives. These concepts also highlight interactions that work against narrative, such as scattered treatment events and fragmentation of care. Narrative theory provides an analytic frame for understanding how clinical competence and specialty power is used to "plot" a coherent therapeutic course, to structure clinical time, to instill desire for treatment and to give hope.[2]

Literary theorists have argued that plot provides the underlying structure of narrative, constructing "meaningful totalities out of scattered events," allowing stories to unfold through time (Ricoeur 1981b: 278). Reader response theorists, such as Wolfgang Iser (1978) and Umberto Eco (1994), have focused attention on the activity of "emplotment," on the response of a reader or hearer of a story who engages imaginatively in making sense of a story. Readers try to "uncover the plot" to determine what is really going on, what is likely to happen as the story progresses. Reader and hearer thus construct a "virtual plot" of remembered pasts and imagined futures which shifts constantly as the action progresses. The virtual plot always contrasts with the "actual plot" of the written text (Bruner 1986).

What Paul Ricoeur calls "narrative time" is also a central dimension of all plots. Narratives thus have a necessary temporal and sequential dimension of beginnings and endings, a directionality, an outcome or conclusion that bestows sense on what has occurred (Brooks 1984).[3] Concern about how the story will turn out, about how the present will be seen retrospectively from the vantage of the ending, is present as a structuring quality in all storytelling and emplotment.

I have found these perspectives especially relevant to narrative dimensions of clinical work in oncology and more generally to understanding the care physicians and nurses provide for the chronically or seriously ill.[4] There is an essentially narrative quality to activities that clinicians and patients engage in together, as they seek over time to make sense of an illness and craft a treatment. Clinical narratives, the stories of these activities, assume special importance when treatments are complex and difficult and disease is life-threatening.

The analysis of excerpts from clinical narratives and of the interpretations of narrative work by oncologists and patients included in this chapter address the importance of interactions between patients and their oncologists in shaping what competence means in the practice of oncology. The narrative strategies employed illustrate how oncologists bring the two worlds of medical science and therapeutics to their patients.

CREATING AND INTERPRETING THE PLOT

Physicians are creators as well as "readers" or "interpreters" of clinical stories. They establish a therapeutic plot for patients, as a course of treatment is set in action, and they "read" the unfolding "actual plot" determined by disease process and patient response. Physicians, even within the same subspecialty, hold a variety of opinions about how best to construct appropriate clinical narratives that are "therapeutic," caring, and productive of desired responses from patients. And they struggle with the difficulties of creating endings when their treatments are ineffective and patients face cancer death.

As creators of clinical narratives, physicians also develop multiple and parallel subplots, each tailored to specific audiences and expressed through interactions with specific actors. For oncologists, these include not only professional colleagues and the treatment team, patients, and patients' families, but the oncology research groups and scientific communities to which they belong. The dimensions of temporality and of duration, outcome, and ending, and therefore the construction of narrative time, may differ for each subplot, for each alternative form of the clinical story.

"Emplotting" or "interpreting" the clinical story is also a crucial imaginative response of individuals who are faced with a disease, such as cancer, and with the unfolding experiences of treatment. When patients and physicians initially encounter each other in the clinical context, they embark on the task of creating and negotiating "a plot structure within clinical time, [placing] particular therapeutic actions within a larger 'therapeutic story'" (Mattingly 1989, 1994). In a theoretically important analysis of clinical work, Cheryl Mattingly refers to this interpretive activity as "therapeutic emplotment." Her study of occupational therapists and their patients focuses on the creative elements of "therapeutic emplotment" and on the shaping of patient experience in the therapeutic moment.

Oncologists often speak about patients as "partners" in the therapeutic tasks of decision making, reporting symptoms, and getting through difficult treatments, suggesting an ideal of a jointly developed interpretation of what larger therapeutic story will emerge out of care. Introducing "emplotment" into an analysis of this clinical work draws attention to how the ongoing experience of disease and treatment is created by clinicians and patients as they engage each other and interpret the impact of treatment on disease.

In oncology, the larger therapeutic story is expected to have direction, instill hope, and create desire in patients to move from illness into a treatment regime that is often arduous and lengthy, in many cases toxic, and occasionally futile. Clinical narratives in oncology also have relatively mundane elements: which therapy will be undertaken first, what side effects may be experienced, what the sequence of treatment will likely be, who will carry out the treatment, and where it will occur. More profound questions lurk beneath the mundane (asking of the "actual plot" of disease process): What are the most effective treatment options? How does one choose among multiple possibilities (such as those available for breast cancer today)? Will treatment, in the end, be successful? How does one interpret the meaning of risk of recurrence? Am I (is this patient) a person who can tolerate aggressive (or experimental or salvage) treatment? What will really happen next?

Clinical narratives are developed with these questions in mind and are structured by clinical time—How will various treatments be scheduled? for the mundane; What will happen next? for the future. Yet, these narratives, and therefore the crafting of temporality, are constrained by disease process and progression, by patients' and physicians' worries about prognosis and endings, by questions of what will happen next, and by patients' life time. Oncologists therefore face a unique challenge in crafting therapeutic time, both for the treatment of patients they believe they can cure as well as for patients for whom the outcome is far more uncertain or where treatment is palliative and death by the disease is near certain. The challenge is heightened by the constant transformation of anticancer therapeutics and the continuous emergence of data about the efficacy of various treatment protocols. Institutional inefficiencies also pose challenges to oncologists and their patients, such as the failure of lab reports and mammograms to be placed in charts, and these may also threaten to distort or fragment clinical narratives, disrupting the sequencing of treatment and rendering narrative ineffective.

The following excerpts illustrate selected narrative strategies used by surgical, medical, and radiation oncologists, as they plot a therapeutic course, involve patients in "reading" and "interpreting" the clinical story, and manage clinical time, from the mundane of daily treatment to the extraordinary questions of what the future holds. Patients' reflections about these efforts indicate but a few of the very complex reactions individuals bring to the narrative endeavor and to their worries about silences and ambiguities as well as about the spoken and explicit aspects of the clinical story.

Narrative Strategies

EMPLOTTING THE TEMPORALITY
OF RECOVERY

Crafting mundane therapeutic time, thereby explicitly seeking to shape patients' physical experience of treatment, recovery, and symptoms, is a conscious process for many physicians. One striking example of the conscious designing of recovery was described by a surgeon who cares for many women with breast cancer. Reflecting on the extraordinary changes in length of hospital stay following mastectomies or breast-conserving surgeries since her residency training—from five to seven days to one to two days—the surgeon noted her teaching service "made a conscious effort to go to two days or less and made a program that would make that easier for patients." (Average hospitalization following breast surgery at the time of the interview in 1993 was four days.) She proposed that two important developments in the care of patients made this change possible. The first was to convince physicians that patients could be sent home with surgical drains that they would be responsible for emptying themselves: "This was the main break that let us get patients out earlier." The second was to create expectations in patients that they will be going home in one or two days. The surgeon's enthusiastic understanding of the meaning of clinical and therapeutic narratives led her to recount how she uses physical symbols (small dressings) as well as talk to bring patients to the expectation of rapid recovery from surgery.

I use tiny dressings when I do things. Sort of the same way that "you think you had a small operation so you get better faster." Most women are prepared ahead of time. I tell them the day that we are talking about the operation, "Most women are in the hospital one, maybe two nights, you certainly stay longer if you've got any problems, but most people feel well enough to go home, and in fact they do." What I've been amazed at is which patients beg me to go home after one night when I thought they would be a two-night-stay kind of person.

Later in our interview, as she spoke about the development of a new breast center "to create the best possible care for women" and to plan clinical studies to interface with basic science, she discussed why she believed narratives powerfully influenced patient experience.

It was so dramatic to me when we went from—we tried to organize a program to have people discharged after two days instead of five or six. It was shocking to me when you know just the difference in how you explained it to them ahead of time and telling them what the expectation was, how differently they did. And I do the same operation, the surgery is not that different. There may be a slight difference in how surgeons do things, but it's almost all expectations. . . . "Small dressing, must be small operation, I shouldn't be sick." . . . I think it makes a big difference.

TEMPORALITY AND PAIN

Management of postsurgery pain is the work of surgical oncology and as crucial to the therapeutic process of breast cancer care as the initial surgery. The following segments from a follow-up visit between a sixty-five-year-old woman who recently received a mastectomy and her young surgeon illustrate how symptoms are placed within clinical and physiological time, as the surgeon seeks to "emplot" expectations of recovery and guide the patient's interpretations of pain.

Patient: I have that shooting pain, constantly.

Surgeon: The discomfort that a lot of women will describe as shooting pain . . . that's where the nerves are irritated from the surgery. You have the skin now growing back and settling down on the muscle since there's no breast in between.

P: At night time, right through here, this here—

S: Have you started the physical therapy?

P: Yes, today.

S: That will help loosen up that tightness. [Patient comments on hot showers helping.] Part of what the physical therapy will do will be to help stretch those muscles out so it doesn't keep going into spasm like that. Part of that is, if you feel over here, you have a little tissue here, but this is still swollen, there's still some fluid here which I'll take out now, and until all the healing is done and the fluid is gone, we'll still get swelling. *But there's even less than there was. When I look at you now, this tissue here, there's less than there was a week ago. So I would tell you that it probably will be at least another month or two while that's improving, but it will. It will get down, it will be much less.* If in the long run it still feels like there's extra tissue there, we can take care of that with very minor surgery. But I bet we won't even need to do that.

P: It's fine with me if you do it and get rid of it.

S: But you might not need to. It may settle. There's still a lot of swelling there. So how's the energy?

The surgeon continued to interpret her patient's pain within a time frame of progress (in contrast to the possibility of additional minor surgery), thereby evolving a larger story of recovery rather than of incidental and momentary treatment.

Patient: I'm so sick of pain [laughs].

Surgeon: I know. You have made so much progress, though. I'm so happy you did not have any trouble with infection at all.

P: Just that tightening. Oh God, is that so tight.

S: Mm-hm. Well, it should feel a little less tight now, when I take the fluid out, that makes it so there's a little less pull.

P: Right here. Right here. It's as sore as can be.

S: It's just because all this muscle and stuff was—what we did, your body's used to having a breast there between the skin and the muscle, and now the muscle and skin are healing together, so it'll be like it is up here, where there's muscle and skin right together. And while that healing is happening, the nerves that were cut and *things that are regrowing give you those sensations and the shooting pain and so forth. But it will eventually settle down and not hurt at all.*

P: I hope that's very shortly.

S: It will. *It will take some time. I'd give it another six to eight weeks to continue improving. It'll get better long before then. I think you're better off than you were a week ago.*

P: I'm better today than I have been, really.

S: Now, how far are we from your operation?

P: I think it was twelve or fourteen days ago.

S: A little more than that, I think. . . . Three weeks. Most people I tell to expect to feel uncomfortable for three or four weeks after the operation. . . . Part of that is that's all still swollen, and *it takes at least eight weeks after the surgery for the swelling to go down.* One more piece of tape, just because it's going to want to fall off. And this swelling, this area is much smoother and less swollen.

Pain is thus linked to healing and regeneration signifying repair of the body, even as it is confirmed as the source of severe discomfort.

ULTIMATE QUESTIONS AND LIFE TIME

Emplotting recovery time from cancer surgery is framed in weeks and at most months and contrasts with the ultimate question of what the future holds, of recovery not simply from surgery but from the disease of cancer. These larger issues of life course and endings are often left unvoiced, but in this interaction both patient and physician acknowledge the limits of therapeutic options. These discussions about life span and chances to defy death by disease are carried out in the language of statistics and odds, thereby bringing clinical science into therapeutic activity. The following excerpts occurred both at the beginning of the visit and near the conclusion, sandwiching the more mundane discussions of recovery and treatment "for the moment." The patient opened their visit by telling her surgeon she liked her medical oncologist.

Surgeon: Did you meet her today? Oh good. So she—did she talk to you about the tamoxifen?

Patient: Yeah. She told me—she told me that after fifty, it was just as good, there was only a three percent chance that the—not the radiation, but the chemotherapy would be better than the pill. And you have to decide on how much of a life span you want. I don't want to be sick at eighty. If I have five years, I'll take my five years and enjoy them.

S: And the other thing that she may have been explaining to you is that there's a three percent chance that you would have a longer life span with the chemotherapy than with the tamoxifen. You might have the same—

P: Life span, that's right! They don't know, and it's—

S: And the treatments are very different. With the chemotherapy you have more side effects while the treatment is going on.

P: Exactly. And you go through that for six months. This lump is killing me.

At the end of the interaction, the surgeon returned the discussion to adjuvant therapy, to whether there were reasons to be "worried," and to how she would continue to monitor the patient's status in collaboration with the medical oncologist. The larger story about the possibility for recovery from cancer is returned to the mundane, as therapy is planned for a period of years and expectations about symptoms and side effects are emplotted.

Surgeon: And we did all those mammograms and everything.

Patient: I know, and that didn't show anything.

S: And we're going to keep an eye on that side too. Now did she tell you, did she give you a prescription for the tamoxifen?

P: Yeah, I've got it.

S: And when did she want you to start taking it?

P: Right away.

S: Good. I agree.

P: Twice a day. And then she said that—

S: You'll be on that for at least five years.

P: Well, she said three anyway, but they're making a study whether it's beneficial between three to five. At least three and then she'll see me in three months anyway.

S: I'd like to see you—are you seeing her sooner to have any blood tests, or just then?

P: Just then.

S: I'd like to see you one more time in the next week or two, to see how the fluid is—there's much less than there was last week, so I think I'm too worried about that. But I'd still like to see you. Next time I may not need to drain you. I'd like to see how you're doing with the physical therapy and hear how you're doing. And also you can tell me how you're doing on the tamoxifen.

P: Right.

The possibility for recovery and chances of cure took a different cast in the patient's first consultation with her medical oncologist. The "for the moment" recovery from surgery and the focus on mundane time was unavailable as an escape from the existential questions. Why this struggle of pain and treatment? Would treatment be futile, pain for naught, as it had been for her sister-in-law years before? Why expose one's body to surgery, to toxic chemotherapies, when there appeared scant likelihood of cure? The unsettling refrain was echoed by the patient's husband when he asked, "Why do surgery if there is no way you can save a person's life?"

METAPHORICAL AMBIGUITY AND THE ROUTINE OF STATISTICAL UNCERTAINTY

The following excerpts capture some of the fundamental questions about endings and outcomes, and illustrate the medical oncologist's attempts to draw the patient into an "appropriate" and meaningful therapy, to engage her in "for the moment" care. As the oncologist teaches the patient and her husband about the possibilities and side effects of adjuvant therapy, she leads them at length through the therapeutic impact and side effects of hormonal and chemotherapies. The visit lasted over an hour, very long in clinical time. The excerpts selected highlight the way the physician brought her scientific understanding of the odds of treatment efficacy to her discussion with the patient of life chances. She was direct, frank, and employed statistics interspersed with metaphors. The interaction appeared to the researchers as warm, caring, and personal as the physician shifted from her "educator voice" to that of empathetic caregiver. Recall the patient had told her surgeon she liked her medical oncologist.

Husband: Why do surgery . . . ?

    MD: Well, you're absolutely right. But with breast cancer—let's just focus on this problem at hand—with breast cancer when you have a lump, before you do the surgery you check to make sure it hasn't gone anywhere else. Dr. S. did that. Everything looked good, and that's why she recommended the surgery. *Now the reason you're seeing me here today is because the surgery's not a guarantee. You're already telling me you know that the surgery alone isn't a guarantee that we're going to cure you, but medical treatment may play a role in increasing your chance of being cured, and that's why you're here.*

After reviewing the history of the surgery with the patient, the findings of lymph node involvement ("the reason you are here"), and the bone scan ("good news—no evidence of spread, so, so far, so good"), the medical oncologist tried to lead her patient through the clinical reasoning behind the choice of adjuvant hormonal therapy. Negotiating treatment choice was interspersed with a physical exam, discussions about pain relief, reflections on the horrible cancer deaths and medical adventures of the patient's close kin, and her fear of treatment, but remarkably, not of death itself.

Patient: What are you putting me on? I want to go on a pill, I don't want to go on chemo.

    MD: I hear you. My job is to just tell you what I think the two treatments will do for you, and then we'll talk through it, because I want to make sure you feel you have the facts that you need to make the decision, and that's really what you're doing here today . . .

    MD: There is maybe even as much as a fifty-fifty chance that a little seed has spread in the bloodstream from that original tumor, and maybe somewhere in your body it might show up in the future. . . . *And frankly I'd probably put that as about fifty-fifty.* So if we did nothing else, there's probably only a fifty-percent chance, on average, that you'll still be alive, free of disease, five years from now. And a fifty-percent chance that you won't, so the tumor might have come back someplace . . .

The physician continued with her "seed" metaphor, noting that the spread and growth of cells in other organs is "a very inefficient process" . . . "like throwing seeds on a garden" . . . "and it's like rocky soil." The adjuvant therapy "can quite often kill [those cells] before they get a foothold," and "it's an attempt to help the surgeon cure you by killing these little seeds." Continuing in her educator voice, she gave her patient the reason she should choose tamoxifen "absolutely."

There is no question that tamoxifen is likely to offer you a benefit. How much of a benefit? Well, if you look at the different studies and average it out, if you've got a fifty-percent chance of being disease free in five years if you don't take it, if you do take it, that is probably going to be increased by maybe twelve percent, maybe fifteen percent, but a significant amount. In other words, instead of a fifty-percent chance of being free of disease, you might be up to sixty-five percent, that order of magnitude. A very significant benefit. Enough that basically no oncologist around the country today would not think of giving you tamoxifen. So that's a given. That's an absolute recommendation. The debate right now is not so much whether or not you should take the tamoxifen, but whether in addition you should consider chemotherapy.

The visit concluded after much discussion of chemotherapy (only an additional 3 to 5 percent benefit, perhaps more with newer drugs, but a toxic, "six months" effort), an undesirable choice. As the patient readied herself to leave, confirmed in her choice—"I'll take my chances," "I want to do something reasonable" (i.e., choose the tamoxifen)—she joked to her physician about being placed on the three-to-five-year protocol—"yeah, well at least you give me three to five years!"

Clinical narratives such as these mix metaphors and messages about time. Narrative time shifts from the immediate to the future. And although the future is uncertain, and expressed statistically so, the immediate and mundane have a measure of certainty, of recommendations that are "absolute." These narratives exemplify the joining of the two worlds of clinical science and therapeutic care.

Two research interviews with the patient cast additional light on these clinical interactions and on the patient's participation in narratives in the making. Prior to her visit with the medical oncologist, she told our researchers she "only wanted to take a pill" (tamoxifen) and had already decided against more toxic forms of chemotherapy given the experience of friends and family. In an interview two months after these visits, she recalled that the oncologist frightened her "with all those seeds growing" and decided she preferred to think neither about breast cancer nor about her daily medication.

EMPLOTMENT OF ROUTINE TREATMENT

Oncologists inevitably encounter the uncertainty of time horizons in their patients' lives, as exemplified in the excerpts discussed above. This uncertainty about time leads to specific narrative strategies to focus patients on the routine of treatment that follows surgery. The practice of radiation oncology emphasizes the routine, perhaps even more than in medical and surgical oncology, because treatments are daily and extend over weeks. Yet radiation treatment is regarded by most patients as out-of-the-ordinary, a high medical technology that conveys fearful images, and radiation oncologists believe patients must be convinced that the treatment is not to be feared, that it is not going "to make their bodies glow" or turn them into radiating creatures. Thus, the routinization of treatment has several goals: to gain patient commitment and to alleviate or diminish fears.

Patients, who are often considered "well" by the treatment team because they are usually ambulatory and have recovered from surgery, react in quite radically different ways to the routinizing of their experiences, both during and after treatment. The emphasis on "for the moment" is often fraught with great anxiety for patients as they complete the surgical stages of therapy and seek knowledge of prognosis and certainty about illness course. Yet in clinical observations and in interviews, patients too appear to evoke, participate in, and at times collude in the shaping of narrative and clinical time in terms of immediacy, maintaining an unspoken ambivalence about voicing the effects of treatment on future illness course.

Excerpts from the first conversation following treatment planning between a radiation oncologist and his breast cancer patient illustrate how the clinical tasks for the subsequent weeks are set in a therapeutic time frame and expectations about how the treatment will be inscribed on the body are emplotted and normalized.

Patient: What should I exp—what happens? I mean what's going to happen?

   RMD: What's going to happen to you?

      P: Yeah.

   RMD: Nothing much. I mean, what's going to happen, in the first two weeks you won't notice much at all. Maybe literally nothing at all. You'll hardly notice anything. After about three weeks you'll notice that the skin of the breast gets a little bit red or warm initially, warm to the touch, and then slightly pink, and then slightly red like a slowly developing sort of sunburn, and usually, . . . if everything goes according to plan, that's about all you'll get that's noticeable on the surface. You may also get a little bit of swelling in the breast, but that's all. Again, you won't—you shouldn't really feel or notice anything else. Obviously, as we said before, we are treating a thin layer of your lung, very, very unlikely to be noticed by you as a symptom. The only other thing you might notice is just a mild fatigue. But otherwise you'll probably not notice much at all. You'll be fine. That's what one may expect.

P: Good [laughs].

RMD: So don't let me down.

P: I'll try not to.

After instructing the patient on breast care during radiation, the oncologist continued to focus the patient's attention on the unfolding course of treatment.

RMD: Anything else? Obviously you know the plan for your treatment is five weeks, like you'll have an hour and then the final week for a boost, six weeks in total. And what we need to do is see you once a week on a Tuesday, where we go over any problems there might be, either specifically about the breast or sometimes, generally about anything. Okay?

Patient: Okay. Fine.

Daily treatment regimes and the activities of the radiation therapy team (the radiation oncology nurses and technicians) set the tenor for the clinical experience. Attention to the details of daily treatment, which are hardly trivial for patients, and the focus on technological requirements establish the ground for more significant encounters, when difficulties of course and prognosis may be addressed. One radiation oncologist, who works with a range of patients from severely ill brain tumor patients to lymphoma patients certain of cure, spoke about this aspect of her work.

There is a lot of housework, the boring part of getting people into radiation therapy. All of those little appointments and time schedules and things. All of that occupies the trivial time when you circle around each other perhaps . . . while you wait to talk turkey, to be more explicit about the effects of treatment and course of disease.

Nevertheless, metaphors of housekeeping suggest unremarkable, possibly comforting, and caring activity, without crisis or threat to daily existence, as in the interaction between the radiation oncologist and patient quoted above. "What will happen?" "Not much." The message from oncologist to patient is that treatment can be integrated into the everyday life world. For patients, the matter-of-factness of a treatment team, whether it be in surgery, radiation therapy, or medical oncology, can be disconcerting, for some maddening, especially when patient anxieties and experience of ambiguous side effects are dismissed as medically unimportant. Nevertheless, the routine of treatment draws most patients into an experience of the less-than-remarkable, of comfort, of the therapeutic momentary, of a return to the ordinary, even while they experience anxieties about what the radiation or chemotherapies are doing to their bodies and fear the ultimate outcome of disease. These complex feelings are held simultaneously and are not incompatible.

Patients as Partners in Clinical Narratives

As women review their experiences of surgery and radiation treatment for breast cancer, they speak about the complex feelings inscribed by the clinical narratives crafted by their physicians. One woman acknowledged how she fluctuated between feeling anxious and feeling "cosseted" by the routinization of treatment experience in radiation. When asked what she took from the weekly status checks in radiation treatment, she responded:

It gives me a lot of comfort seeing them [the physicians]. Because I think they're keeping up and they're keeping a check. And the odd thing is, during my initial meetings with any of the doctors, I felt so cosseted and warm and cozy, and then as the days went on I got nervous again. I felt like somebody was sort of cosseting me and taking care of me and putting me under their wing, like everything's going to be all right. And then as soon as I left, I was fine, elated and fine. Then as days wore on, it's like I can't wait to get back to MGH to know I'm going to be all right. So I think . . . it's very, very good for people to meet with doctors once a week. It makes you feel they care enough about you.

Another patient recounted how her feelings kept changing as she entered the routine of radiation treatment.

I think that in the beginning, when you're very fragile, is the time when you really want people to pay attention. Now coming in here, I was terrified. Even though I knew I wasn't going to feel anything and, coming in for the first three or four treatments, I would cry through the whole treatment. And everybody just talks over you, they don't pay any attention, because what . . . everybody must do that. Now I come in, "Oh, thank God I'm here." You really can get into a routine. So I think that in some ways the routine of it all helps you to accept it more.

Later in the interview, the patient expressed her fears of radiation, and how these fears become routinized and unacknowledged even while the routine of treatment has a comforting side.

I actually enjoy coming here in a way, because—you're on the other end for a while. But you go in and it's, they're talking over you, and all of that's fine, but you want them to pay attention. You really want somebody to keep hold of your hand. I mean once you get into routine, you don't care if they even— I mean, I like a little hello, how are you, and we have a little joke and all that. But the first couple of days, I felt very fragile. And I would have liked it better if people acted like something was about to happen to me. Because it was. Something was happening, and all I could think about was those movies, you know, the radiation movies, Hiroshima and all that stuff, and you're thinking, "Oh my God, they have all this—my poor little body." And I'm thinking, "Well this is going to help you."

Contrasting radiation treatment to her experiences with the process of diagnosis, a third patient referred to it as "the most benign treatment I have ever had in my life." The patient went on to praise one of her physicians for

giving me permission to feel lousy . . . that it was okay for me to feel tired, because everybody I've talked to who's had radiation said, "Oh. Hey it didn't bother me at all! I felt like really Superman all the way through the whole thing." I'm falling all over myself and coming over and putting my head down between my legs, going "Oh my God, I'm a wimp." . . . I shouldn't need permission, but I did need permission to feel lousy from the radiation, and she gave it to me. You need permission to feel.

PATIENTS AS READERS

Patients, just like physicians, are "readers" as well as partners in the creation of the treatment narratives in which they engage with physicians, nurses, and therapeutic teams. Most women interviewed in our breast cancer study attend to the "plot" they believe is being shaped for them by their oncologists, often with heightened sensitivity. They interpret not only the treatment routine, the daily actions, the chitchat or lack thereof, the physicians' caring or distancing concern, but even changes in the length of the sounds of the radiation machine as it delivers its rads to their bodies. The comings and goings of the radiation technicians are also monitored, as fears of being "forgotten" with the machine left on, or the radiation technician somehow becoming incapacitated and unable to turn the machine off or making an error, surface. Patients acknowledge these are irrational fears, but they still have them.

As they seek to discern what the likely effects of radiation will be upon their bodies "in the moment," these women also seek to interpret the multiple plots that their bodies, their medical teams, and the disease have in store for them. They become acutely aware of the silent as well as vocalized reactions and comments of their physicians, nurses, and technicians; what they attributed to views of their medical team in the interviews with researchers were not necessarily discussed with either their nurses or physicians. And even though most patients engage in frank discussions with their oncologists at some point during treatment of the likelihood of cure, recurrence, or uncertainty of prognosis, the clinical narratives that are created in daily clinical time appear to have at least as great a significance in creating overall therapeutic experiences for patients as these discussions about ultimate outcomes. Thus, clinical narratives shape patient experience not only during treatment but long after the conclusion of a treatment course when treatment is viewed retrospectively.

Individuals' reactions to the narrative emphasis on "for the moment" has been variable, both positive and negative. Some women interviewed several months after completing radiation therapy experienced "radiation rage" or anger about the "unsaid." Routinization of experience, dismissal of symptoms of fatigue, and lack of explanation about what was "really happening" to one's body in response to radiation were among the complaints. Others felt more comfortable, and regarded the experience as positive and their physicians as benign and competent. A few patients actively avoided retrospective readings of the clinical story as they sought to unencumber themselves from illness, to "get on with their lives."

Integrating Two Worlds: Scientific Uncertainties and Standards of Care

The competent practice of oncology is deeply influenced by the rapid transformations in the bioscience of cancer and the production and marketing of experimental protocols and new treatments. Oncology, like other high-technology specialties, epitomizes a particular genre of contemporary medical culture, one in which competence and caring are joined in the technical act and in the plotting of the technical course—a series of linked technical acts. The oncologist's construction of a competent and caring clinical narrative, in part through the emplotment of a series of technical acts, must respond to these transformations and the uncertainties inherent in the clinical science of the specialty. Patient expectations also shape how clinical science is integrated into therapeutic narratives as well. This is particularly evident in breast cancer treatment, where many patients are knowledgeable about changes in the surgical treatment of the disease (the introduction of breast-conserving surgery) and aware of the hormonal, chemo, and bone marrow transplant therapies introduced over the past decade.

"RULES CHANGE"

The reflections of two clinicians on recent changes in breast cancer treatment—that of a medical oncologist and a surgical oncologist, a woman and a man—evoke the changing nature of clinical standards and clinical science and its impact on how clinical narratives are shaped.

The medical oncologist, who had worked with breast cancer patients for over ten years, spoke about how communicating with patients changed over the past "seven or eight years" as "the rules changed" and everything became more "complicated" as therapeutic options expanded. Nevertheless, her philosophy of patient care fit well with these changes:

As I wrap up the sessions with my patients, I usually remind them that what I've been trying to do is to be their educator. I tend to approach my patients with "We're a team, and my job is to make you aware of the facts you need to know to make your own decisions." And then I spend time going through what I think about where they are with their disease. "Here's what you have, here's how I interpret it, here are the prognostic factors, and therefore this is what I think your options are." And then I go through what I think of the different options. But ultimately, I want them to choose what they do. Now it depends on who your patient is and where they come from as to whether they are comfortable with that or not. I would say that maybe seventy-five percent of my patients are comfortable with that. They like the idea that they're making the decisions and they're in charge. And then maybe one in five . . . basically says to you "Well you're the doctor, what do you think?" . . . And that's okay too. It's refreshing sometimes to have someone not want to ask all the questions, but that's not really my view of how health care is or should be right now, and it's certainly not what most women with breast cancer are looking for.

The oncologist compared the less inquisitive patients from her early years of training with women today. "Most women are very well educated now, they've heard all the buzz words, and . . . they've read enough that they want to ask all sorts of things." And although patients are more informed today and physicians are now legally required to inform patients about therapeutic options (in Massachusetts), she attributed these changes in communication with patients to new discoveries in the bioscience and therapeutics of breast cancer. Her reasons are interesting:

Well, the therapies have been proven to be beneficial. When I was a fellow, it was not quite clear who did and who didn't benefit from chemo. . . . I would say ten years ago we were beginning to understand that the benefits were more likely to be reserved only for the younger women, and that was sort of blessed in the middle of—1985—with an NIH consensus report. . . . So the rules were easy. And the patients would walk in and you'd be able to—anyone could do the same analysis and you knew what that patient would walk out with. Well, the rules over the last seven, eight years have gotten much more complicated, not only with—they're now coming out to say that the older women do benefit from the chemotherapy, but also lymph-node negative women may benefit, and maybe a combination of chemo and hormonal therapy is better than either one. And then, they've come out with all these different prognostic factors that may push you to give chemo in someone that you would have thought originally would have been in too good a prognostic group to need chemotherapy. So suddenly it becomes very complicated.

A noted surgical oncologist—"I operate all over the body"— echoed the increasing complexity of the clinical rules and standards of care in breast cancer treatment.

Obviously breast cancer patients used to be very easy to take care of when I was an intern in 1970; everybody got a mastectomy, that was basically it—it was easy. And often they came in and had a breast biopsy done, and if it was positive, we just went ahead with the mastectomy and there wasn't a lot of discussion about it. And now that there are so many options, it takes a lot of time. I wouldn't call it a dilemma, but the hardest part, probably, is helping your patient decide what they're going to be comfortable with, because it's not always what you might—right out of the starting blocks—think would be necessarily what their decision would be. But then as you kind of draw things out and talk about their social situation . . .

MEDICINE ON THE EDGE

The current controversy over bone-marrow-transplant treatment for metastatic breast cancer exemplifies difficulties in deciding what constitutes a competent clinical narrative, given changes in clinical science and the dynamics of formulating clinical standards. It also poses an ethical dilemma both in terms of societal and individual costs, both financial and personal. As a medical oncologist noted (in 1993), this expensive "salvage therapy" has had dubious therapeutic credentials, and in recent clinical trials patients who initially responded positively to transplants "were all relapsing at six or eight months after the transplant." Yet in 1994 some patients sued for insurance coverage for these treatments, and some oncologists encouraged their use. Although the cost of providing bone marrow transplants has declined dramatically as treatment shifts from hospital to outpatient services, the therapeutic efficacy remains questionable. Guiding patient choice in the face of complexities in the clinical science of oncology therefore emerges as a fundamental challenge to the specialty's clinicians (in contrast to its scientists). As the bioscience of the field expands and decisions to choose competing therapeutic options become ever more complicated, especially given the uncertain efficacy of many treatments, the task of joining the two worlds of oncology and creating competent clinical narratives that work against inappropriate or fragmented care looms larger.

CHAPTER NINE

Epilogue

The Relevance of Competence to Policy

In this final reflection, I consider the relationship between social and cultural studies of professional competence and policy research. The quote from a recent medical graduate—"What do we care about? 'What do we care about?' is the hardest question in all of medicine"—requires even more consideration in this era when the American medical commons is in turmoil. As American society once again confronts the inequities in health coverage and resources and the daunting rise in the cost of health care, the essence of medicine *as a profession* at times becomes overshadowed. It often appears from our public discourse that "what medicine cares about" is economic self-interest, cost containment, or, in the best light, the organization of health services.[1] Certainly, the current social and cultural environment appears to many of the profession's most notable scholars and commentators as the antithesis to good doctoring in the clinical context and as a momentous challenge to our society's institutions of health care.[2]

How we conserve the medical commons—our institutions of patient care, of medical education and training, of bioscience and clinical research, and even of the engineering and production of medical products—depends in large measure on how we, as a society, preserve and continue to produce the *profession* of medicine and the allied health professions. The various ways we conceptualize and create physician competence stand at the heart of this task.

Two themes developed in the book bear upon our understanding the culture and political economy of contemporary medicine and its relevance for health policy for the medical commons. The preceding ethnographic studies on malpractice and obstetrics and reviews of the national scene illustrate how "competence" provides a medium for articulating relations of power and competition for resources (prestige, money, control over knowledge) in clinical practice, training, and research. Second, competence as a symbolic domain not only draws together widely diverse meanings and social contexts but must be disaggregated if we are to discern and judge the social uses competence discourse bears.

Physician Competence and Political Economy

When doctors are popularly perceived as granting priority to their personal finances and cost containment rather than to patient well-being (Eisenberg 1992; Relman 1980, 1992), it is not remarkable to assume that claims to medical competence (or disparaging the competence of others) are driven by the economic and political interests of individual physicians, of specialty groups, or of particular institutions of health care. Current policy debates on health care reform employ discourses on quality of care and physician competence to argue both for and against universal health coverage. Those favoring reform note the difficulties the poor and rural populations have in gaining access to competent doctors and quality medical care (Weinstein 1994). Those opposed argue that universal health coverage and managed care organizations will undermine the high standards of competence for American medicine, and will diminish the care most Americans receive. As the teaching hospitals and medical schools lobby the national government for consideration of their special financial needs in the health reform bills, they justify their requests in terms of the competence and quality of the profession and its foundation in the biosciences.[3] It is no surprise that just as curricular and specialty battles are fought out in the language of competence and quality, current debates over health care reform, especially as shaped by the medical profession, are carried out in similar language and through similar discursive actions. In such scenarios, the meaning of physician competence becomes infused with the political economy of professional viability and competition, and with questions about the future organization of medical work. Identifying links between discourses on competence and the profession's economic interests has become part of our society's everyday commentary on medicine.

It is far less common, however, for our popular discourse on the profession to attend to how our cultural assumptions about physician competence profoundly influence the political economy of our health care system. This link between the culture of competence and the political economy of practice is particularly apparent in specialties such as oncology and in "the political economy of hope." The relevance for other high-technology medical specialties is evident. In spite of concerns about containing health care costs, our society expects that American physicians (oncologists, other specialists) will knowledgeably offer patients the latest anticancer therapeutics and treatment "weapons" as part of the clinical task of instilling hope and carrying out treatment, even while acknowledging and balancing the danger and risk of these "weapons."[4] These activities designate in large measure what Americans mean by clinical competence in oncological practice in the United States today. What we conceptualize as good medicine—*what we think medicine should care about*—from the utilization of new biomedical knowledge and techniques to the crafting of therapeutic narratives for patients, has far-reaching consequences for our society's investment in designing, producing, and marketing therapeutics, as well as in the organization of health care.[5]

The analytic model I proposed (figure 1, page 175) links the clinical to the societal, the culture of medical practice to the larger political economy of biomedicine. Although I emphasized clinical narratives in oncology in this discussion, the model also suggests additional directions for research in the sociology and anthropology of biomedicine. Comparative studies of biomedicine reveal that clinical practice occurs in local worlds, that medicine's "scientific universalism" remains in tension with local cultural and economic constraints, and definitions of competent medical practice and what lies at the essence of "physician competence" vary enormously (M. Good et al. 1993; M. Good et al. 1994).[6] The specific cultural foundations, historical developments, and political economies of biomedical practice not only construct what is meant by physician competence, but influence how treatment narratives are framed and therapeutics are chosen. For example, the way in which physicians convey information about diagnoses and prognoses and choose treatment options for patients varies even across societies that commit vast resources to high-technology medicine, as is evident in comparisons among the United States, Italy, and Japan (see note 6). Nevertheless, local cultures of biomedicine are neither isolated nor distinct from cosmopolitan medical culture. Dominant biotechnical societies, such as the United States, export not only medical knowledge, through direct training, scientific discourse (publications, meetings, international clinical trials), and medical products, but also a culture of biomedical practice. A global perspective is essential if we are to understand and evaluate what physician competence means, including the choice of therapeutics and the organization of health care, in our own society.[7]

Disaggregating Physician Competence

The facets of physician competence I have discussed thus far emphasize both discourse and narrative analyses as ways to understand how medical competence is negotiated through interaction in different contexts of professional power—from medical education and primary care medicine, to high-technology specialties such as oncology. In this final discussion, I reconsider three dimensions of meaning carried by this core symbol as they bear upon future directions for research and implications for health policy. These are empirical competence, competence and clinical narratives, and competence as an essentially contested domain. I conclude with a note on competence in international perspective.

EMPIRICAL COMPETENCE RECONSIDERED

Although physician competence is a symbolic domain, it clearly refers to an empirically definable set of practices that are grounded in knowledge of the basic biosciences and lie at the very heart of what our society and the profession mean by good doctoring. Concern over what constitutes "empirical competence" attracts a good deal of attention from the profession's educators and moral philosophers. As one longtime physician educator remarked to me, "the discourse on competence serves to organize thought and develop skills that result in medical expertise in an objective and real sense."[8] Nonetheless, when physicians try to specify exactly what these skills and knowledge are (what constitutes this medical expertise), this seemingly certain empirical domain appears enormously complex, nuanced, and far less precise.

Recent programs designed to define essential competencies for physicians who will practice into the twenty-first century exemplify the complexity and slipperiness of this domain.[9] The Robert Wood Johnson Foundation Commission on Medical Education began a study in 1990 in response to what it called "a perception of many medical educators that medical student education needed fundamental change" and "thorough reform" (Marston 1992:1144). Although this call echoes those of earlier and even ancestral generations of medical educators (Ludmerer 1985; Morgan's "Discourse" from 1765, in Merton, Reader, and Kendall 1957),[10] the contemporary efforts address the extraordinary advances in molecular medicine, the challenge posed by "the new biology," the changing social contexts in which medicine is practiced, and potentials for lifelong learning. The Johnson Foundation Commission report emphasizes *processes* rather than discrete and specific *content* as essential to educating competent physicians. Stressing the integration of biological and behavioral sciences in medical practice, the commission argues that the culture of medical schools must be designed to instill professional values "that embrace integrity, a recognition of the limits of physicians' competency, and patient trust" and lauds the potential of "the science of medical informatics" (Marston 1992:1145). The report also calls for continuous *and* interdisciplinary evaluations of educational programs and trainees and discourages reliance on medical board exams (tests of discrete components of medical knowledge at the end of the second and fourth years), long held as the hallmark of achieved professional status. Although not new, the recommendations are radical, critical of professional traditions.[11]

Clearly, we see in the Robert Wood Johnson Foundation Commission report more than simply a reformulation of assumptions about the definition of competence from discrete knowledge bits to an ongoing process of learning and evaluation. Although this shift fits with contemporary understandings of the social processes of medical education, the Commission has embarked on a pursuit to not only redefine empirical competence for physicians for the twenty-first century but reshape relationships among the various basic science and clinical disciplines. Thus, in the guise of reforming medical education and in the language of professional competence, the Robert Wood Johnson

Foundation has cast a wider net to tackle the very structure of medical school hierarchies and relationships across basic science and clinical departments.

The Pew Health Professions Commission project also illustrates just how "imprecise" the meaning of empirical competence may be. The Pew group listed seventeen "competencies" for "future practitioners" (O'Neil 1992); the list is wide-ranging and illustrates the group's intent to have a broad impact on inequities in American society that go beyond traditional formulations of clinical competence. The Pew report uses the language of competence in medical education to write health policy and to propose ways in which changes in the health care system might be carried out through institutions of medical education. Whether such an approach confounds many of the central issues of medical education or whether it enhances thinking about how our society trains its physicians and thereby provides quality medicine for all segments of the population remains an open case.

An agenda for research on social innovation is suggested by these two examples, among others, on medical educational reform. How will new cultures of medical competence be shaped by such projects? Does economic power translate into cultural authority among medical school faculties? Will commission reports and foundation funding from philanthropies such as the Robert Wood Johnson Foundation, the Henry J. Kaiser Family Foundation, and the Pew Trust influence investments in the new biology, in "medical informatics," and even in the social and behavioral sciences? Will such projects encourage the restructuring of departments in the basic sciences, as recommended? How will this bear upon the meaning of competence in the biosciences? Upon the content of new bioscience knowledge? Will the context of clinical training shift, from tertiary care hospitals to ambulatory and primary care clinics, as recommended? What social uses—such as the power struggles among disciplines of the biosciences and clinical medicine—are carried by discourses on competence in medical education?[12] In a review of contemporary innovations, the foundations currently appear as primary actors.[13]

These examples illustrate how "empirical" competence becomes a vehicle of influence and power in the culture of biomedicine. Social studies of reform in the more narrow scope of medical education open an analytic lens to broader transformations in contemporary biomedicine, from organizational changes in the disciplinary context in which knowledge is produced (e.g., the disappearance of anatomy departments and the rise of molecular medicine) to how knowledge is taught and institutionalized in clinical practice.

COMPETENCE AND CLINICAL NARRATIVES

When physician competence is considered in terms of clinical narratives rather than as a specific set of skills and bounded body of knowledge held by individuals, the analysis shifts to ongoing clinical activities. Interactions between students and the training hierarchy, between doctors and their patients, as well as among groups of physicians, become of paramount importance.

Competence in the creation of clinical narratives focuses attention on how clinical knowledge is used to select and negotiate a clinical course, at times to persuade both patients and other clinicians of the appropriateness of treatment, of a course of action. As illustrated by the studies of oncology, clinical narratives frequently include the framing of time with the goal of instilling hope. When narratives are well crafted, treatment decisions and the experience of disease may be placed within the overall life course of patients. The management of uncertainty about medical science and disease course remains a major task in the creation of competent narratives, and working with a changing data base and with what is ultimately unknowable becomes part of the clinical challenge.[14]

Studies of competence in clinical narratives also bear upon health policy and the continuing education of health professionals. Analyses of clinical narratives suggest ways to evaluate specialty practice beyond the gross data of "good" or "bad" outcomes, beyond longevity, cure, and palliation, to examine whether narratives are integrated or fragmented, whether they are fraught with mismanagement. Given that many patients are subject to extended treatment, a practical consequence of conceptualizing medical "competence" in terms of the quality of clinical narratives provides physicians and treatment teams with ways to critically assess what they are doing over time. Such a formulation asks not only *how* but *how well* technological actions are wed to clinical stories and the integration of care? Having physicians attend to the structure of narratives, through educational seminars and reviews, offers one additional way to teach and enhance clinical competence.[15]

A second policy-relevant issue emerges from attention to the narrative dimension of how physicians guide patients in therapeutic choices and frame time through the experience of treatment. Pressures on the organization of care may impact upon and perhaps erode the competent management of time in clinical narratives, especially when physicians are discouraged from investing in this patient-centered activity. Irrational practices and inefficiencies of health care organizations can also lead to the disruption of clinical narratives. Even minor systems-level failures, such as the loss of films and records, violate the therapeutic endeavor, often leading to expensive as well as personally troubling fragmentation of care. Establishing health care settings that highly value competence in clinical narratives may reduce the emotional and financial expense of fragmentation.

COMPETENCE AS A CONTESTED DOMAIN AND ITS SOCIAL USES

A third dimension of competence links the social context of medical knowledge and practice and historical moments. Unprecedented advances in the biosciences and medical technologies characterize medicine in our contemporary world, and thereby create a fluid and shifting base for standards of clinical practice. As procedures and therapeutics move from categories of experimental to routine, as what is accepted as "empirical" knowledge changes with new discoveries from the sciences basic to medicine, clinical practice comes under review. However, new knowledge and new "certainties" are not necessarily nor easily transferable to clinical medicine (as illustrated by research on "risk assessment" in obstetrics; see chapter 5). And the routines of clinical practice (such as the use of electronic fetal monitoring) are often altered with difficulty, even in light of successive studies that question the value of particular modes of practice. When uncertainty of therapeutic efficacy is introduced (as in the choice of particular anticancer therapies), formulating clinical practice standards, and thereby definitions of clinical competence, is bound to pose difficulties for competing groups within the profession.

"Turf battles," such as those between specialists and generalists in primary care and among competing specialty groups or institutions, are often barometers of these shifts and developments in medical knowledge and techniques. Such contests are not only indicative of power struggles within medical hierarchies (over which group has the right to authorize knowledge and to establish standards of practice) but also highlight alternative ways in which medical knowledge is interpreted in clinical practice and claims to medical competence and specialty power are framed.

Research on *competence as an essentially contested domain* has explicit policy implications for the profession and for its regulators. As attempts are made by government and medical educators to reverse the ratio between primary care physicians and specialists in American medicine,[16] the ethics of specialist-generalist relationships should be continuously reviewed. Research on "competence"—on its social uses and multiple meanings—may not only provide a critical analysis of these relationships and thus further social studies of the medical profession but also suggest policy guidelines for managing specialty turf battles, for contributing to the development of clinical practice guidelines, and for fostering the appropriate integration of advances in the clinical sciences into clinical work, at both the primary care and specialty levels.

Studies of the multiple meanings and social uses of "medical competence" also focus our attention on medical liability and the malpractice crises of the past two decades. As medical liability policy is reviewed and our tort laws reevaluated, the linking of judgments of physician competence to patient compensation requires continuous rigorous evaluation. The Harvard Medical Practice Study (1990; and Weiler 1991; Weiler et al. 1993) is but one step in this direction. Findings suggest that disaggregating patient compensation for adverse events and medical negligence from judgments of physician competence may be socially if not financially more beneficial to patients and the public. Whatever developments unfold in the domain of tort law and malpractice reform, the gritty issues of evaluating competence and incompetence in medical practice (as well as carelessness and negligence) will continue to loom large for the professional community as well as for the public.[17] Mechanisms for peer *and* public review, for affirming the responsibility of professional collectivities, and for meaningful quality control of medical practice will continue to benefit from a critical examination of the various social uses, contexts, and meanings of "physician competence."

COMPETENCE IN INTERNATIONAL PERSPECTIVE

When "physician competence" is regarded from a comparative cross-national perspective, the diversity of biomedical cultures becomes extraordinarily evident; such diversity has been created through historical, economic, and political circumstances that are local as well as cosmopolitan. Again, research and policy may be pursued through comparative studies of medical competence, to link the culture of clinical practice to the political economy of medicine. In particular, the exploration of clinical narratives highlights this link and the ethical dilemmas it poses, especially in societies where resources are far scarcer than in the industrialized world.[18]

Similarly, examining the relationship among modes of practice and ideologies of caring provokes questions about the influence of the international medical marketplace on conceptualizations of physician competence. When competent medical practice is defined in terms of spending two minutes per patient "writing" prescriptions and proliferating the use of pharmaceuticals, when making psychiatric diagnoses takes the form of offering C-T scans from the latest MRI machine purchased for a for-profit private clinic, when an act of caring includes choosing inappropriate antibiotics for diarrheal disease to assuage parents' expectations, then training in biomedical competence faces economic as well as ethical constraints. As biomedical competence is considered globally, the local contexts of market and entrepreneurial medicine within which so many physicians throughout the world practice must also be addressed. Many doctors with whom I have spoken in Asian and African countries talk about the discrepancy between their medical knowledge (they regard themselves as competent in terms of the knowledge they hold in their heads) and their medical practice. Although often counterindicated by their knowledge, practices are adjusted to the market, to the struggle to be financially viable. Practices are also tailored to local cultures of patient-physician relationships, to clinical circumstances, and ultimately to the scarcity of institutional and/or patients' resources.[19] When the care of patients on an obstetrics or internal medicine ward means controlling the spread of HIV, and sterile facilities, even latex gloves, are in short supply, then medical competence must be regarded in the context of extreme scarcity. Educational and institutional policies must be shaped in accordance with these exceptional circumstances and the ethical dilemmas they pose.[20] What may be unquestioned "competent" standards of medical practice in a society of riches may appear impossible to achieve in a context of scarcity.

Nonetheless, in many societies of the world, the profession of medicine is highly regarded, and the brightest of university students are directed into or choose to practice medicine. The field is often financially lucrative and brings prestige to individual physicians in many countries. Given the enormous investment in medicine (and sometimes in health) by individual patients, families, and governments, scarcity of resources does not absolve the medical profession from maintaining practice standards, quality patient care, and an ethically conscious stance. In fact, the universal ideals of biomedicine, as it is taught and at times practiced around the world, appear to emphasize "competence," "knowledge," and "skill," as well as a form of bioethics that bridges local and cosmopolitan cultures of caring for patients, even in the face of the power of the medical marketplace.

Comparative analysis of the culture and organization of biomedicine across societies should highlight not only universal aspects of medical work and of bioethics but also the economic constraints on medical competence. When we consider the medical commons both globally and nationally, the problem of limited resources is hardly confined to the third world. How costs and profits of therapeutics bear upon the conceptualization and teaching of medical competence requires close consideration; what is considered to be "good" medicine may be economically driven. Such analyses should help us conceptualize "competence" as a category for research relevant to policy as we continue to study and produce the profession of medicine in the twenty-first century. In terms of policy, they lead us to pursue the question of how the culture of biomedicine should be shaped in the future, of "what medicine should care about" both locally and globally.

Notes

Introduction

1. See Paul Starr's *The Social Transformation of American Medicine* (1982) for an elaboration of the idea of cultural authority and Eliot Freidson's classic work *The Profession of Medicine* (1970b) for an analysis of the sources of the profession's cultural authority. See also Freidson's more recent or updated essays in *Professional Powers* (1986) and *Medical Work in America* (1989).

2. Howard Hiatt introduced the notion of the "medical commons" in "Protecting the Medical Commons: Who Is Responsible?" in the *New England Journal of Medicine* in 1975, portending the political and popular concerns of nearly two decades later. He wrote:

> Surely, nobody would quarrel with the proposition that there is a limit to the resources any society can devote to medical care, and few would question the suggestion that we are approaching such a limit. Yet there is almost universal recognition that among the additional demands that must be made on our resources are those designed to address the current inadequacy of medical care for large sectors of the population. The dilemma confronting us is how we can place additional stress on the medical commons without bringing ourselves closer to ruin. (1975:235)

Hiatt raised these concerns when U.S. health care expenditures amounted to 8.3 percent of the GNP; by 1994, we were spending approximately 14 percent of the GNP on health care. See also Brennan 1991.

3. Throughout my field research projects, the national malpractice crisis of the 1980s intensified, profoundly influencing how physicians spoke about medical incompetence. At a forum on the changing malpractice climate, several clinicians questioned whether physicians themselves were not contributing to the malpractice crisis by their willingness and ready availability to become "expert witnesses," to "break the conspiracy of silence." One remarked he "had

personally found it appalling that we had moved from what was perhaps not an entirely ideal situation of a 'conspiracy of silence' to a position where members of the faculty are testifying against each other and not always on very solid, intellectual or professional grounds." Shortly after the forum, a document from a major teaching hospital in the area recommended departmental chairs review credentials of staff physicians called as expert witnesses in malpractice cases.

4. My emphasis on "American" medicine, rather than medicine or bio-medicine, is deliberate, because national cultures of medicine have particular characteristics, even when they have global reach. Eugenio Paci (1993) notes that in Italian primary care medicine, the battle to make competence more central to the work of doctoring was lost in the 1970s. Nevertheless, local physicians in Italy are beginning to experience challenges to local practices from cosmopolitan medical centers such as those in Milan (and the United States) that seek to impose standards of practice generated from these centers of biomedical research and clinical trials.

Chapter One

1. See Byron Good 1994 for a discussion of Bakhtin (chapter 7) and semantic analysis in medical anthropology; also our earlier work, including M. Good 1985, and B. Good and M. Good 1980, 1981.

2. Freidson identifies the rank-and-file practitioners; the teacher-researchers who produce knowledge, define standards, and establish criteria for credentials; the professional managers who allocate resources; the "visible scientists"—that is, influential professionals who speak for the profession; and the professional associations that represent corporate interests (1986:211–215).

3. See Charles Bosk's critique of work that dominated medical sociology in the 1960s and 1970s and the characterization of the profession of medicine in largely monolithic terms (1979).

4. See Weiler 1991:2; Campion 1990; Weiler et al. 1993 for figures on malpractice and claims.

5. IOM 1989a,b; ACOG 1985, 1988, 1990.

6. See Relman 1989:97–99; Brennan 1991. Popular laments made their way into the nation's press throughout the 1980s and into the 1990s. A recent example includes "Wariness Is Replacing Trust between Healer and Patient," by Gina Kolata, *New York Times,* February 20, 1990 (A1 and D15). In the middle 1980s, many physicians found fault with the legal system, as exemplified by a letter written to the *New York Times* by James Sammons, M.D., executive vice president of the AMA, titled "The Crisis Is Not in Medical Care, but in our Legal System" (February 23, 1986, section IV, p. 20, late city ed.).

7. See James Holzer's excellent overview (1984; reprinted in Campion

1990) of the meaning of "risk management," a "relatively new administrative intervention" in health care (1990:195). Originally "coined by the insurance industry in 1963" to refer to controlling loss in business activities, it came to medicine in the 1980s. Holzer argues there was a shift in focus in meaning from its original use in business because of its link to professional concerns for patient safety.

8. The aims of the JCAHO "Agenda for Change," according to James Todd, executive vice president of the AMA, were to "create standards that provide a foundation for continual quality improvement activities within health care facilities, establish performance monitoring indicators, and improve assessment of the facility compliance with JCAHO standards. The Agenda also calls for the development of 'clinical indicators of quality' to enable better analysis of the quality of patient care" (Todd, in Campion 1990:xvii).

9. See Weiler 1991:46, 56, 63, 71, 116–117, 122, 135, 177 n. 23.

10. The Harvard Medical Practice Study (1990), primarily noted for its finding that one in one hundred hospitalized patients suffer medical accidents or adverse events due to negligent care, also included a mail survey of 739 physicians and in-depth interviews with 47 physicians. These smaller studies were designed to elicit how physicians experienced the tort system and whether they regarded it as a deterrence to medical negligence. Although the findings are ambiguous about deterrence capacity, these two small studies allowed physicians to point out what they regarded as flaws and inequities. The comments made in response to the in-depth interview (as well as the survey responses) resonated with my own studies of physicians, and with letters and commentaries published in the professional medical literature during the same period.

11. Discussions with Lynn Peterson (a surgeon and ethicist), Anne Lawthers (a health service researcher), and Troyen Brennan (a lawyer and internist) brought out this interpretation.

12. Holzer notes that "most physicians have learned that an adverse clinical outcome is not, by itself, sufficient grounds for a malpractice action" (Holzer 1990a:82).

13. See Weiler 1991, Campion 1990, and IOM 1990 for discussions of these efforts from legal and medical perspectives. Hendricks Garnick and Troyen Brennan (1991) note that "26 physician organizations have developed over 700 practice parameters while another 150 are forthcoming," and that in 1989, Congress endorsed these efforts, creating the Agency for Health Care Policy and Research "to develop, evaluate, and disseminate practice guidelines" over the next five years (2857). However, a current review of very limited evidence led the authors to suggest:

The direct influence of practice guidelines on the number of malpractice suits is probably limited because the development of detailed guidelines is in an early stage and a one-to-one match does not yet exist between the medical conditions now addressed by practice guidelines and the causes of claims. (2859)

See also Lomas et al. 1989 for a discussion of changing physician behavior.

14. The casebook is an example of a highly focused professional discourse,

designed for practicing clinicians, for residents, and for those who teach and train physicians. Its purpose is to aid rank-and-file physicians (and their teachers in Continuing Medical Education and residency programs) to understand and cope with medical liability problems.

15. In contrast with medical malpractice cases that address the momentary negligence or medical accidents of individual practitioners, risk management focuses on collective knowledge and practices and on the responsibility of the professional *collectivity,* often defined by specialty, seldom by locality. The shift from local to national definitions of standards of care and from a definition of the professional collectivity from local communities of physicians to the national community of specialists was in part encouraged by the demise of the "locality rule." This rule held that a physician's actions would be judged by the standards of the medical community—or similar communities—where he or she practiced. The shift from the local to the national has in part been driven by the liability crisis of the 1980s, and in part by organized medicine's efforts to exert its power nationally. Holzer notes that the demise in the 1970s of the "locality rule" and the replacement of local measures of medical practice standards with national ones have led to the emergence of "a new perspective on clinical standards" (1990a:82–83).

In 1985, a rural physician commented that he perceived a looming change in who bore responsibility for the competence of individual physicians who were granted hospital privileges; responsibility was becoming the domain of the local hospital's privilege-granting body, the medical staff. He regarded the change with dread; the malpractice climate led him to move from the community in which he had successfully practiced for a number of years. Assuming responsibility for the *collective* competence of the community's medical staff, particularly during a period of discord and strife over what constituted competent and authorized medical practice, appeared potentially hazardous—financially, professionally, and emotionally.

Peer review can be threatening, especially in light of the devastating results of the Patrick case, in which an antitrust suit was brought against physicians involved in the peer review process in a small medical community. See Weiler 1991 and Campion 1990 for useful discussions of peer review, medical staff responsibility for the collective competence of providers, and the impact of the Patrick case. The advent of nationally published standards may address these issues.

16. Categories of clinical standards include those which are "voluntary/physician generated standards; involuntary/underwriter-generated standards; or statutorily imposed standards" (Holzer 1990a:84).

17. Freidson, in reviewing the move toward employment rather than entrepreneurial enterprise of many physicians, reminds us that "the position of individual professionals has no necessary bearing on the position of their professions as corporate bodies" (1986:129).

18. I thank John Stoeckle for drawing my attention to and giving me Savage's book, *A Savage Enquiry.* The parallels to the crises I had observed in rural America were striking.

Introduction to Part I

1. The ethnographic research in Coast Community was a joint effort by my husband, Byron Good, and myself. It was partially funded by two grants from the National Institutes of Mental Health to examine rural primary care practice and physician recognition of and response to psychosocial problems of primary care patients (NIMH Grant MH16463, 1980–83, research directors M. and B. Good; NIMH Grant MH39532, 1985–85, P.I. M. Good, Co-P.I. B. Good). See M. Good, B. Good, and Cleary 1987. As part of these ethnographic and clinical studies, communities from the Health Systems Agency California District I (district authority was abolished under the Reagan administration) were visited and physicians and other health providers and administrators were interviewed. The agency district extended to the area north of Sacramento and Santa Rosa and ranged west to east from the Pacific coast to the Nevada and Oregon state borders. It included coastal, valley, foothill, and mountain terrain, much isolated and rugged. Other communities in the region were visited as part of conflict-resolution work for Health Systems Agency I and as part of a study funded by the University of California on the viability of rural hospitals in northern California. During these consulting and research visits, hospital administrators, nurses and hospital workers, physicians, and community members were interviewed and group meetings attended. More intensive ethnographic and clinical research on primary care practice was carried out by our research team in a total of seven rural medical communities representing the diversity of the district.

Chapter Two

1. "Local medical docs" (abbreviated as "LMDs") is a term used for community physicians by some university-affiliated residents and faculty. The status of community physicians changed in recent decades as residency training became more common and the financial picture of health care services altered. During the past decade, community physicians were regarded as important sources of referral for tertiary care centers competing for patients. Community physicians were also courted through lucrative Continuing Medical Education programs sponsored by institutions of academic medicine. Rural physicians can maintain contact with the medical meccas in their regions through CME programs, referral networks into metropolitan and academic medical centers, and board certification.

2. One community in our rural primary care study had the good fortune to have a choice between two physician-owned hospitals from 1930 to 1954. In the oral histories we collected, people recalled how the physicians who practiced at one hospital would impugn the competence of those who practiced at the other hospital. These discussions were not confined to professional

colleagues but included patients and the public. It was considered "fair game" if not gentlemanly to compete through comparing the competence of rival physicians. Talk about competence clearly characterized rivalry among physicians, even prior to the "coming of the specialists."

3. Through our collection of oral histories, it became strikingly evident that high physician turnover has historically plagued many remote rural towns in the Northwest. Given the economic and malpractice context of contemporary American medicine and the stresses on rural hospitals, it appears that specialist-generalist rivalry may contribute to the fragility of rural medical communities even as standards of medical competence and patient care are improved.

4. My students and I carried out smaller research projects in rural and urban New England in the mid-1980s and found many simmering conflicts between specialists and generalists, especially over the practice of obstetrics. Inter-physician rivalry was expressed through public as well as professional critiques of the competence of colleagues in communities in Maine and Vermont and in Boston.

5. Among the many studies of birthing and obstetrics, a recent contribution from medical anthropology is Robbie Davis-Floyd's *Birth as an American Rite of Passage* (1992).

Chapter Three

1. A contemporary gender joke that was making its way through medical circles played on this image. "A man and his son are traveling at high speed along a super highway. They have a serious accident and are taken to the emergency room of a major medical center. The chief surgeon on call, upon entering the exam room to see the man's son, turns to the resident on duty and says, 'I cannot treat this patient; he is my son.' How is the son related to the surgeon?"

Chapter Four

1. See Sally Falk Moore's discussion of processual anthropology and the analysis of events as diagnostic of larger societal processes (1987), and Clifford Geertz's discussion of Karl Mannheim and Harold Garfinkel's contributions to "the documentary method" (1965: 153–154).

2. Gender politics can also erupt within a specialty. A conflict similar to the crisis of competence that took place in rural America was unfolding in the mid-1980s in London between male and female obstetricians (Savage 1986).

3. Areas of disagreement include whether family practice physicians should deliver breech births, use forceps, deliver twins; whether an obstetrician must

be present when a patient is given oxytocin; whether women who have previously had Caesarean sections should be allowed to be delivered vaginally by family practitioners. Gray areas include debates over who should give prenatal care and attend births of high-risk patients. The issue of home births, and family practice involvement in home births, continues to be a source of contention. Most family practice physicians, including those who practiced home births in the past, currently avoid home births because of difficulties with obstetrical consultant coverage and medical liability insurance.

4. JCAH is the Joint Commission of Accreditation for Hospitals, a state regulatory agency.

Chapter Five

1. The American Bar Association recommended rejecting early proposals from the AMA to restrict malpractice suits. The ABA contended that "the medical profession, in seeking changes in the tort law system, has shown a willingness to trade away the rights of individuals in the hope of easing a perceived burden on itself" (*New York Times,* February 4, 1986: "Lawyers-vs-Doctors Battle on Malpractice Builds," A1, A21).

2. The crisis for obstetrics took place in a context of wider changes in the medical profession which disturbed many physicians. See the 1988 *Milbank Quarterly* issue titled "The Changing Character of the Medical Profession" (vol. 66, no. 2). Articles by John McKinlay, John Stoeckle, Donald Light and Sol Levine, and Vincente Navarro present contrasting interpretations of the state of the profession in the late twentieth century, from proletarianization (McKinlay) and loss of professional autonomy, to restratification and the persistence of professional autonomy, although reconfigured. Stoeckle examines the decline in passion and sense of mission in medicine. This cultural transformation is viewed as disheartening for the individual physician and detrimental to the profession's moral and cultural core.

3. In 1970, 49 residency programs were established; by 1986 there were 381 programs, many based in community hospitals rather than in medical school teaching hospitals, thereby marking the less "academic" nature of the specialty.

4. The rise in the number of physicians coincided with the emergence of mid-level primary care clinicians who had a degree of practice independence. Certified family nurse-practitioners, nurse-midwives, and physicians' assistants added to the scope and breadth of primary health care teams.

5. The Southern, Mid-Atlantic, and lower New England states traditionally have been most hostile to family medicine obstetrics, in contrast to the Pacific, Western, and Midwestern states; within the same region, family physicians in rural practice were twice as likely to practice obstetrics as those in urban areas (Schmittling and Tsou 1989:183). The ratio of obstetricians to population was also significantly associated with family physician attrition from obstetrical practice in the 1980s (Kruse, Phillips, and Wesley 1989:600).

6. By comparison, in 1989, 33 percent of first-year residents in internal medicine and 16 percent in surgery were women.

7. See ACOG 1988:5, 11, table 36.

8. Only 52 percent of all suits brought against OB/GYNs were for obstetrical cases (ACOG 1988: tables 20 and 21). Thirty-one percent of obstetrical suits were for neurologically impaired babies (table 21).

9. Michael Klein and his colleagues introduced the notion of "endangered species" and used it to describe the threatened state of obstetrics in family medicine in Canada (Klein et al. 1984).

10. The concerns of academics were echoed by the community of family physicians as well. See "Letters" to the *Journal of Family Practice* 29 (1989): 361, 443, 604, 606.

11. Klein argues that the discrepancy between theory—i.e., low intervention birthing—and practice even within most family medicine practices is extensive and argues against the "mini-obstetrician model" for family medicine (letter to the author, Nov. 16, 1993).

12. William Arney contends that after World War II, the profession of obstetrics began to reformulate its concept of pregnancy from "a segmented to a processual phenomenon, from an entity characterized by a demarcation of normal from abnormal to one with a natural course and quantitative deviations from it" (1982:138). The concept of the continuum in modern obstetrics has thus confounded the efforts to define "high-risk" and "low-risk" patients and practice. See also Gifford 1986 for an analysis of the semantic domains of risk in breast disease.

13. Programs in risk management covered many fronts in obstetrical care. Virginia developed a no-fault compensation policy for cases involving neurologically impaired babies. Maryland offered a plan to set premiums per delivery, thus enabling physicians with small obstetrical practices to contain liability costs. In Minnesota, a risk management task force chaired by a family physician and made up of obstetricians and family physicians developed nonclinical risk management guidelines "intended to address some of the most common, preventable problems that contribute to patient injuries and jeopardize the defense of birth-related malpractice claims" (Minnesota Medical Insurance Exchange 1988:567).

14. In 1987–88, Scherger organized a program in California for ninety family physicians with the goal of developing risk management guidelines to evaluate whether they would lead to a decline in malpractice claims, premium costs, and litigation anxieties (Scherger 1987; Scherger and Tanji 1988).

15. Nelson reported 99.6 percent of those with meconium staining did not go on to suffer from cerebral palsy. Meconium was present in 18 percent of all births surveyed; 98 percent of infants with bradycardia below sixty beats per minute who survived did not later have cerebral palsy. 98 percent of infants who had cerebral palsy had no indicators of major asphyxia, a claim not accompanied by supporting data (Nelson in Ryan et al. 1989:58–59).

16. Professor of Health Policy at Harvard Medical School and the Kennedy School of Government, a pediatrician and former surgeon general under President Carter.

17. Arney (1982) argues that the specialty of obstetrics has been historically grounded in clinical experience rather than in clinical research; Allan Young, referring more generally to clinical practice, suggests "scientific standards are simply inappropriate in clinical settings given over . . . to making decisions where clinical evidence is incomplete or ambiguous" (1981:382).

18. A recent study (Brennan, Hebert et al. 1991) found that Medicaid patients were less likely to sue their physicians than other patients.

19. Barriers to specialty obstetrical care were documented in an analysis of over forty-six thousand medical birth records from 1982 to 1984 in the state of Maine (Onion and Mockapetris 1988). Family physicians or general practitioners were proportionately more likely to provide birthing services to Medicaid and uninsured patients than were obstetricians, particularly in urban areas with the greatest density of obstetricians. Board certified family physicians, more comparable to their obstetrician colleagues, were also less likely to provide obstetrical services to poor patients than physicians not board certified. Because "more patients in these higher risk groups are delivered by family physicians and osteopathic physicians" and because of the late involvement of consultants for complicated deliveries, the finding "probably understates what is likely even greater redistribution of poor patients away from obstetricians" (1988:425).

20. In the early 1980s, reimbursement for obstetrical services for Medicaid patients in states as diverse as Maine and California was often insufficient to cover the cost of malpractice premiums. In Maine during the period of the Onion and Mockepetris study (1988), total reimbursement amounted to $300 per patient. In California, during the crisis in Coast Community, state reimbursement per patient was $480.

21. Roger Rosenblatt recommended collaboration with nurse-midwifery to define new paradigms for obstetrical practice in family medicine (1988). Midwifery is rarely mentioned in the *Journal of Family Practice*. The less-than-enthusiastic response to Rosenblatt's suggestion is indicative of serious competition posed by midwives whose practice turf is similar to that of family physicians. In addition, nurse-midwives frequently work for obstetricians and are part of the specialty's competitive edge.

22. Although alternative birthing programs are often staffed by midwives, obstetricians have been involved in their creation and are generally central to their continuation and success (see the discussion of the Coast program in chapters 3 and 4).

23. See Arney 1982:146–147 and chapter 7; see also Davis-Floyd 1992.

24. In 1990, one in four women who gave birth was single. The obstetrics patient population is characterized by older prima previa patients and by adolescent, often poor and single, patients.

25. See AMA/ACOG 1987; AMA/AAFP 1988; Robertson 1988; IOM 1989b; Petersen, Reiss, and Wadland 1990.

Introduction to Part II

1. Our previous publications on this study include M. Good and B. Good 1989; B. Good and M. Good 1993; and B. Good 1994.

2. Twenty-four students from the class of 1989 entered the first New Pathway class; the remainder followed the traditional curriculum, known as the classic pathway. We followed the class of 1990 most systematically, including twenty New Pathway students, twenty-two classic pathway students, and eleven students from the joint program between Harvard Medical School and Massachusetts Institute of Technology. In addition, students from 1989 and 1991 classes were interviewed throughout their bioscience and clinical education. In all seventy-two students participated in the study. We were assisted with interviews and analysis by anthropology graduate students, Eric Jacobson, Lindsay French, and Karen Stephenson; Margaret Zaldivar assisted with transcribing.

3. Michael Klein (Professor of Family Medicine, Vancouver, B.C.), noted that

Canadian medicine viewed the McMaster experiment with great suspicion and the graduates . . . were judged very harshly, often considered 'less competent.' . . . It probably took 10–15 years to rebalance the situation, so that McMaster graduates are now considered to be at least as good as the graduates of most medical schools in Canada. One might believe this involved not only the passage of time but the redefinition of competence throughout the Canadian medical scene. (Letter to the author, Nov. 16, 1993)

4. NOVA produced and aired two shows on the New Pathway, following the class of 1991 through the four years of Harvard Medical School: "Can We Make a Better Doctor?" (Episode 1521, December 1988) and "So You Want to Be a Doctor" (Episode 1812, November 1991).

5. This comment was made at a continuing medical education conference by Dean Daniel Tosteson and is drawn from my notes of the discussion.

6. See Marston 1992. The Robert Wood Johnson Foundation is supporting educational innovations in a number of American medical schools, encouraging rethinking the integration of the biological and clinical sciences and training. See chapter 9.

7. The Robert Wood Johnson Foundation, the Henry J. Kaiser Family Foundation, and the Pew Foundation among others have recently invested in new programs and medical education innovation. See Marston 1992 and Primary Care Task Force (AMA) 1992:1092–1094.

8. As in earlier eras, the critical professional and public discourses about medical training and practice continue to influence training innovations; they also play a role in how our institutions of medical education seek and justify public investments in the production of physicians. Leaders of Boston area medical schools and teaching hospitals made a special plea to President Clinton and his health reform team to give special financial support and consideration to institutions of medical training and research in devising a government plan. The groups also offered support for the administration's health care re-

form efforts. See *New York Times,* March 21, 1994: "Clinton Offering Medical Centers a Compromise" (section B, p. 7, late city ed.).

Chapter Six

1. See Derek Bok 1983. Gordon Moore, a general internist, spearheaded the practical aspects of the New Pathway, assisted by other committed faculty, including Susan Block, a psychiatrist who developed the patient-doctor curriculum, and Dan Goodenough, a basic scientist who headed the New Pathway's Oliver Wendell Holmes Society.

2. Although the source of the "classic" naming is obscure, it was no accident that it occurred at a time when the Coca Cola's company's efforts to change its formula led to a popular outcry and the marketing of the traditional formula as "Classic Coke."

3. Medical students from Kansas interviewed in the late 1950s (see Becker et al. 1961), medical students at McMaster in the early days of the school's innovative case-based curriculum (see Haas and Shaffir 1991), and medical students at LaVal in Quebec in the late 1980s (see DesMarchais 1991) fret over "what they need to know." In the first two years of the New Pathway innovation, Harvard's "classic" curriculum students often touted that they "knew" what they needed to know (at least in the preclinical courses), in contrast to their New Pathway colleagues who, while perhaps receiving more favors and greater investment of faculty time, did not know what they needed to know. The contest between the two groups during the preclinical years often was expressed in this language of knowing.

4. Although New Pathway students initially experienced hostile comments and aggressive surveillance on occasion from faculty and residents who were dubious about their educational "experiment," questioning usually abated as students proved themselves through their performance. As the New Pathway became the common pathway in preclinical education for all Harvard Medical School students, the faculty and deans turned to reform the clerkships and to teach residents and faculty attendings New Pathway educational methods and ideology. They acknowledged that influencing the culture of clinical training is a formidable task given the numerous teachers (residents and attendings), the demands of the teaching hospital for service, and the organization of the training hierarchy. Power resides not in the medical school but in the departments of the various specialties; thus incremental changes and persuasion were used to address resistance. Innovative clerkships in ambulatory care and maternal-child health attempted to institutionalize New Pathway values into the clinical context, as did a third-year patient-doctor curriculum.

5. See Hunter 1991 for an interesting literary analysis of narratives in medicine, especially chapter 3, and Crabtree and Miller 1991; see also Kleinman 1988b and M. Good et al. 1990 for accounts of patients' illness narratives.

6. Few points were earned for complete social histories or assessment of

psychosocial status. This was ironic given the emphasis placed on various versions of the "biopsychosocial model" in the first two years of both the New Pathway and the classic curriculum's longitudinal Introduction to Clinical Medicine. One faculty member, a longtime participant-observer of medical education, remarked that "Psychosocial content is not just neglected, it is systematically downgraded!" He noted that students who show interest in the psychosocial aspects of medical care are labelled "psychosocial jocks" and "closet psychiatrists."

7. The etymology of "fascinoma" comes from "fascinating" and "oma" as a medical ending; thus, a medically intriguing and fascinating case. A "zebra" is a rare, unusual disease, just as zebras are rare in comparison to horses (in North America).

Chapter Seven

1. Highly regulated, formal and informal interactions between medical students and faculty, residents, and interns lead students to develop a sense of clinical competence and a professional identity with physicians above them in the hierarchy, with "mentors" and "role models." These processes of professional socialization have generational continuity—and they are discussed by students, residents, and faculty physicians in their daily talk—as well as in the academic literature on medical education. Robert Merton and colleagues, in their classic study of medical education in the 1950s (*The Student-Physician,* 1957), argued that professional socialization occurs through identification with faculty physicians; in contrast, Howard Becker and colleagues posed student culture against professional and faculty culture, and thus the title of their project, *Boys in White* (1961). This debate influenced subsequent work on professional socialization, particularly in medicine, but has largely been put to rest as more recent studies by scholars such as Donald Light (1988) incorporate both perspectives.

2. In *Boys in White* some graduates reportedly wished to enter solo and rural practice as a means for escaping the surveillance of others in the profession. This option is not readily available today because of changes in peer review procedures, the increased density of physicians, the demise of solo practice, and the rise in group and HMO practices in which professional colleagues hold a financial as well as professional interest in a colleague's competence.

3. *Competence Considered* (Sternberg and Kolligian 1990) brings together recent theorizing by psychologists and psychiatrists on competence throughout the life cycle. Albert Bandura (pp. 315–362) argues that a judgment of competence is a social construction and that performance and self-efficacy are major concepts in psychological analyses of personal competence. Kolligian also notes "the surprising ease with which contextual and social factors can convert competence into incompetence" (347) with consequences for the "impairment of future performances" (347). Kolligian refers to this as "the plasticity of incompetence." Although my emphasis is on the production of a

cultural construct, the current psychological theorizing on competence helps to explain why "performance" and the variability of evaluation is so important to medical students in training. These papers are innovative in that competence is not seen as a state, a set property of an individual, but rather as socially produced.

4. See Bosk 1979 for a detailed analysis of learning surgery through mistakes and errors.

5. See James Scott 1990. Scott's analysis of discourses of the powerless examines the many ways "resistance" to the domination of the powerful is constructed. Interpretations of illness symptoms as modes of resistance of the powerless has been taken up by several authors in medical anthropology as well. See Margaret Lock 1990:250 on Greek immigrant women in Canada and Aihwa Ong's (1987) *Spirits of Resistance and Capitalist Discipline: Factory Women in Malaysia*. The concept of "resistance" in medical education is of course of a different order and magnitude; even as relatively lowly members of the privileged educated elite, students can hardly be regarded as oppressed, regardless of the personal experiences that lead some to intermittently feel this way. Nonetheless, students experience speaking out against sexism or racism or defending their patients as resistance against a powerful, hegemonic order.

6. "GOMER" is a term of disparagement for unfortunate patients, often alcoholics or people who are homeless, who live on the street, but it is also used for older, less competent patients. It is an acronym originally meaning "get out of my emergency room," that is, "GOMER."

7. Activities such as the evolving ethics program incorporated into third-year patient-doctor tutorials at Harvard should expand opportunities for students to develop a professional moral voice during the course of their clinical training. See Branch et al. 1991.

Introduction to Part III

1. Michel Klein (letter to the author, Nov. 16, 1993); Taylor 1988.

2. See M. Good 1990; M. Good et al. 1990; Lind et al. 1989; Lind et al. 1991 for discussions of earlier studies of American oncology at tertiary care centers. For comparative cross-cultural studies of the culture of oncology in the United States, Japan, Italy, and Mexico, see M. Good et al. 1993; M. Good et al. 1994; Gordon 1990; and Hunt 1992. M. Good 1994, *Medicine on the Edge*, explores the clinical and scientific worlds of late twentieth-century oncologists. Previous studies of the culture of American oncology included interviews with over fifty surgical, medical and radiation oncologists associated with teaching hospitals, observations of clinical work in radiation and medical oncology, and a study of fifty-five patients receiving radiation therapy.

3. I thank the Cummings Foundation for supporting the project Clinical Narratives and Breast Cancer (grant to the Center for the Study of Culture and Medicine, Harvard Medical School, Cummings grant P.I. Arthur Kleinman, project P.I. Mary-Jo D. Good). Collaborating oncologists include Rita

Linggood, Irene Kuter, Simon Powell, and Barbara Smith. Susann Wilkinson and Maria Carson interviewed and followed patients, taped the clinical interactions, and engaged the clinical staff. Martha MacLeish Fuller has transcribed the interviews and clinical interactions with great care. Mary Adams assisted with the literature review in the early formulation of the project. The cooperation of the clinical and clerical staff at Massachusetts General Hospital, including Robin Delaney, Mimi Bartholomay, and the radiation technicians allowed the project to move forward. Special thanks go to the oncologists who generously participated in the study and to the patients without whom the project would not have been possible.

4. Regional variation in the promotion of new therapeutic protocols still exists and may be linked to legislation. For example, geographic variation in the use of breast-conserving treatment was identified by researchers in 1992 (Farrow et al. 1992, Nattinger et al. 1992). Researchers noted that the analysis of national Medicare data in 1986, for women 65 to 79 years of age, indicated "substantial variation among the states in the proportion of women with local or regional breast cancer who underwent breast-conserving surgery." Breast-conserving surgery ranged from a low of 3.5 percent in Kentucky to a high of 21.2 percent in Massachusetts, with Massachusetts, New York, and Pennsylvania significantly above the national mean (P 0.001) and eleven states, including Minnesota, Wisconsin, Nebraska, and seven Southern states significantly below the mean (Nattinger et al. 1992:1103). This difference may be due in part to the medical culture of a region and in part to legislation, although the two are clearly linked. Massachusetts requires physicians to discuss all surgical options for breast cancer with patients—that is, mastectomy versus breast-conserving surgery, with and without radiation and adjuvant hormonal therapies and chemotherapies.

5. *New York Times,* March 28, 1994: "Litigious Patients Lead Insurers to Pay for Unproven Treatments," by Gina Kolata, A1, A11, late city ed.

Chapter Eight

1. Holland 1989; Lind et al. 1989; Love 1991.

2. Studies of physician-patient interactions, using discourse or conversation analysis, have greatly contributed to our understanding of power between professionals and patients in clinical encounters. See Mishler 1986a; Todd 1989; Waitzkin 1991, among others. My analysis of narrative should be distinguished from these forms of conversational/discourse analysis.

3. Peter Brooks speaks of plot as "the design and intention of narrative," of "what shapes a story and gives it a certain direction of intent of meaning," a logic developed through "temporal sequence and progression" (Brooks 1984:xi).

4. I thank Cheryl Mattingly for our dialogues on narrative analysis as applied to clinical work; these conversations led me to interpret what I was observing in my work in oncology in new ways. See Mattingly 1989, 1994.

Mattingly, in her remarkable study of occupational therapists and their patients, introduced the notion of "therapeutic emplotment" to analyze what takes place in clinical interactions between patients and their caregivers. I have taken up her insights about emplotment to highlight how oncologists shape patient experience through "emplotment" in clinical narratives.

Chapter Nine

1. Leon Eisenberg, among others, has lamented what is envisioned as a disturbing and dismaying trend (see also Stoeckle 1988; Relman 1992). Eisenberg sounds a moral warning to the profession:

The lexicon of our hospitals is rife with terms borrowed from the corporate world; teaching hospitals "market" and "demarket" (rid themselves of money losing clinical services), diversify, "unbundle," "spin-off" for-profit subsidiaries, develop "convenience-oriented feeder systems," maneuver to adjust case mix, and triage admissions by their ability to pay. (Eisenberg 1992:10)

Eisenberg calls for the profession to "strive to the utmost to maintain our traditional fiduciary role" and argues that the essence of that role is that "the doctor's fundamental moral obligation is to use her knowledge and her skills for the good of the patient" (1992b:9).

2. Julius Krevans, Chancellor of the University of California at San Francisco, fears an overemphasis on economics in contemporary discourse on medicine and writes:

The student who learns medicine in an environment where the bottom line is cash flow will become a different kind of person than someone educated in an environment where, whether we do it or not, we at least hold out that the bottom line is the satisfaction of patient's needs. . . . [If physicians] become less committed to a profession and have less understanding of the public avowal embodied in our calling . . . the next generation and the generations to come will be the losers.

3. See "Clinton Promises Changes in Health Plan to Aid Medical Education," by Adam Clymer, *New York Times,* March 21, 1994, A1, late city ed.

4. See "Litigious Patients Lead Insurers to Pay for Unproven Treatments," by Gina Kolata, *New York Times,* March 28, 1994, A1, A11.

5. The recent expansion of bone marrow transplantations for the treatment of various metastatic cancers, including metastatic disease from breast cancer, is but one example. Current estimates by local medical oncologists of cost per treatment run from approximately $150,000 to a far more manageable cost of $25,000 to $50,000. The argument of tertiary care hospitals introducing these treatments, and therefore treatment units and specialists designated to carry out these therapeutics, is that as more patients are offered this treatment, the costs will decline dramatically. See note 4. See also David Mechanic's discussion of the questionable efficacy of much of our medical technologies (1994: chapter 1).

6. The particularity of the wedding of the culture of competence with the

political economy of medical therapeutics is highlighted when we compare American and Japanese medicine. When Japanese physicians treat cancer patients, they frequently mask the diagnosis of cancer; maintaining silence or ambiguity about the disease has until very recently been regarded as essential to good and competent medical practice. Until recently, the treatment of choice for many Japanese physicians was Krestin, a Japanese-produced anticancer drug; it had no toxic side effects, yet it also had no scientifically proven efficacy. Research oncologists from the Japanese National Cancer Institute have recently been highly critical of the use of this drug and the practice of nondisclosure, thereby initiating a redefinition of medical competence in the practice of oncology. In 1989, the Japanese government recommended that Krestin be used only in conjunction with other anticancer chemotherapies or where no effective treatment has been identified. Krestin held the largest market share of anticancer therapeutics in Japan in the 1980s (Swinbanks 1989a, 1989b. See also M. Good, Hunt, et al. 1993 and M. Good, Munakata, et al. 1993 for a fuller discussion of the Japanese example. See M. Good 1990; M. Good, Hunt, et al. 1993; M. Good, Munakata, et al. 1993; Gordon 1990; Hunt 1992 for additional comparative studies).

7. Physicians "generate about 75% of all costs incurred in the provision of health care services," although services provided by physicians per se only amount to approximately 20 percent of total costs. Medical and surgical therapies, diagnostic procedures, and hospitalization account for the rest (Eisenberg 1992).

8. Leon Eisenberg, memo to the author, July 29, 1993.

9. See Marston 1992; Marston and Jones 1992; O'Neil 1992; and the Report of the Medical Schools Section Primary Care Task Force, AMA, JAMA 268: 1992; see also Enarson and Burg 1992:1141.

10. See Enarson and Burg 1992:1141; Martini 1988.

11. In 1985, Harvard Medical School formed a task force to devise new ways to augment and perhaps replace the National Boards as a measure of professional competence of graduating students. The difficulty of this task was recognized in the failure of the committee (members included highly regarded clinicians and educators) to devise a replacement for the National Boards exam.

12. The Robert Wood Johnson Foundation spent over $20 million in an effort to restructure medical education and redefine the essence of medical competence in the training context. Twelve schools received planning grants of $150,000 each, and eight schools were each awarded $2.5 million to undertake new educational programs. A five-year study of the impact of this endeavor on the various schools is being carried out by a research team led by Gordon Moore.

13. The foundations in collaboration with many medical school faculty produce a joint discourse on reform and innovation. Nevertheless, faculty resistant to change find projects such as those funded by the Robert Wood Johnson Foundation to intrude on the "independence," "traditions," and "freedoms" of the academy. But most faculty see innovation as essential given the major changes both in the biosciences and context of medical practice.

The push toward raising the prestige and power of general medicine is one goal fostered by the foundations, in particular by RWJ. Many within medicine have also championed this goal as they urge ways to redress the generalist-specialist imbalance and fret over the disappearance of the generalist (Colwell 1992; Moore 1992; Petersdorf 1992).

14. When the scientific quality of clinical trials is questioned because of scientific fraud or sloppiness, as in the recent studies of breast cancer treatment (the use of tamoxifen, breast-conserving surgery, and radiation treatment), treatment choices become even more difficult to evaluate, as recently reported in the press: "Fraudulent Breast Research Places Burden on Cancer Field," by Richard Knox, *Boston Globe,* March 31, 1994, p. 1, morning city ed.; "U.S. Halts Recruitment of Cancer Patients for Studies, Pointing to Flaws in Oversight," by Lawrence Altman, *New York Times,* March 30, 1994, B8, late city ed. These reports were followed by reactions in the medical journals (Angell and Kassirer 1994; Bernier 1994; Bivens and Macfarlane 1994; Broder 1994; Fisher and Redmond 1994; Huet 1994; *Journal of the National Cancer Institute* 1994; Poisson 1994; Rennie 1994; Richer 1994).

15. Current seminars on clinical narrative and the reflective practitioner include oncologists and medical students engaged in the breast cancer project and prove promising.

16. See Primary Care Task Force (AMA) 1992:1092–1094. Congress has also proposed a policy that would reduce federal government loans (HEAL) available for medical students in those schools which have fewer than 50 percent of graduates selecting primary care residencies.

17. In press stories in August, 1993, it was reported that the Clinton administration's health care planning task force proposed that patients should sue the organizations that employed their physicians rather than individual physicians per se for malpractice or negligence, thus placing the burden for regulation and oversight of practice on the corporate collectivity. This formulation by a government task force continues the general shift from individual to collectivity for assuring and regulating medical competence.

18. Many physicians interviewed expressed distress over having knowledge about but limited access to biotechnologies, screening capabilities, and new but expensive treatments for diseases such as cancer. Disclosure of information about treatment options is political and moral in the context of scarcity and societal inequities. Should patients be told the "efficacy" rating of their drugs? Should increased longevity be assessed and conveyed to patients, who may be utilizing scarce family resources not for cure but for palliation and only a brief extension of life? These ethical difficulties are met with passionate distress, even as physicians may personally benefit from the importing of the latest technologies and chemotherapies (M. Good, Hunt, et al. 1993:205).

19. At times physician competence includes political action such as when caring for patients means buying food for those incarcerated in hospitals (as reported by Ana Ortiz [1994] for psychiatric hospitals in the Dominican Republic), or placing one's life in danger by caring for patients during civil strife. See Gani et al. 1991 for a discussion of an analysis of discrepancies

between physicians' knowledge and prescribing behavior in the treatment of acute diarrhea in children in Indonesia.

20. My colleagues, who were practicing physicians on the faculty at Muhimbili, estimated that in 1991, 60 percent of patients on the internal medicine wards and 10 percent of obstetrical patients on the OB wards at Muhimbili Medical Center/Hospital in Dar-es-Salaam, Tanzania, were HIV positive.

References

AAMC/SSS (Association of American Medical Colleges Section for Student Services)
>   1992   *Facts: Applicants, Matriculants, and Graduates.* Washington, D.C.: Association of American Medical Colleges.

ACOG (American College of Obstetricians and Gynecologists)
>   1983, 1985, 1988, 1990 Professional Liability and Its Effects. Reports from Surveys of ACOG's Membership for the years 1983, 1985, 1987 (reported in 1988), 1990. ACOG, Washington, D.C.
>   1985   Standards for Obstetric-Gynecologic Services, 6th ed. ACOG, Washington, D.C.
>   1989   Standards for Obstetric-Gynecologic Services. 7th ed. ACOG, Washington, D.C.
>   1992   Annual Report of the American Board of Obstetrics and Gynecology. Data on Specialty Profile provided by ACOG.

Adelstein, S. J., and S. T. Carver, eds.
>   1994   *New Pathways to Medical Education: Learning to Learn Medicine at Harvard.* Cambridge, Mass.: Harvard University Press.

Adler, Valerie
>   1990   Faulting the Medical Malpractice System. *Harvard Public Health Review* 2 (1): 20–29.

AMA (American Medical Association)
>   1988   *Specialty Profiles, Obstetrics* (chapter 8). Chicago: AMA.
>   1993   *Physician Characteristics and Distribution in the U.S.* Chicago: AMA.

AMA/AAFP (Council on Long Range Planning and Development in Cooperation with the American Academy of Family Physicians)
>   1988   Council Report: The Future of Family Practice. *Journal of the American Medical Association* 260:1272–1279.

AMA/ACOG (Council on Long Range Planning and Development with the Cooperation of the American College of Obstetricians and Gynecologists)

1987   Council Report: The Future of Obstetrics/Gynecology. *Journal of the American Medical Association* 258 (24): 3547–3553.

Angell, Marcia, and Jerome P. Kassirer

1994   Setting the Record Straight in the Breast-Cancer Trials. *New England Journal of Medicine,* May 19: 1448–1449.

Annandale, Ellen

1989a   Proletarianization or Restratification of the Medical Profession? The Case of Obstetrics. *International Journal of Health Services* 19 (4): 611–634.

1989b   The Malpractice Crisis and the Doctor-Patient Relationship. *Sociology of Health and Illness* 11:1–23.

Anspach, Renee R.

1988   Notes on the Sociology of Medical Discourse: The Language of Case Presentation. *Journal of Health and Social Behavior* 29: 357–375.

Arms, Suzanne

1975   *Immaculate Deception: A New Look at Women and Childbirth in America.* Boston: Houghton Mifflin Co.

Arney, William Ray

1982   *Power and the Profession of Obstetrics.* Chicago: University of Chicago Press.

Bakhtin, Mikhail

1981   *The Dialogic Imagination: Four Essays by M. M. Bakhtin.* Edited by Michael Holquist and translated by Caryl Emerson and Michael Holquist. Austin: University of Texas Press.

Bandura, Albert

1990   Conclusion: Reflections on Nonability Determinants of Competence. In *Competence Considered,* ed. Robert Sternberg and John Kolligian. New Haven, Conn.: Yale University Press.

Becker, Howard S., Blanche Geer, Everett C. Hughes, and Anselm Strauss

1961   *Boys in White: Student Culture in Medical School.* Chicago: University of Chicago Press.

Bernier, George M., Jr.

1994   Fraud in Breast Cancer Trials. Correspondence. *New England Journal of Medicine,* May 19, 1994: 1461.

Bivens, Lyle W., and Dorothy K. Macfarlane

1994   Fraud in Breast Cancer Trials. Correspondence. *New England Journal of Medicine,* May 19, 1994: 1461.

Block, Susan D., and Gordon T. Moore

1994   Project Evaluation. In *New Pathways to Medical Education: Learning to Learn Medicine at Harvard,* ed. S. J. Adelstein and S. T. Carver. Cambridge, Mass.: Harvard University Press.

Bok, Derek

1983   *President's Report 1982–83.* Cambridge, Mass.: President and Fellows of Harvard University.

Bosk, Charles
   1979   *Forgive and Remember: Managing Medical Failures.* Chicago: University of Chicago Press.
Bowman, Marjorie A.
   1989   The Quality of Care Provided by Family Physicians. *Journal of Family Practice* 28 (3): 346–355.
Branch, William T., Ronald A. Arky, Beverly Woo, John D. Stoeckle, Donald B. Levy, and William C. Taylor
   1991   Teaching Medicine as a Human Experience: A Patient-Doctor Relationship Course for Faculty and First-Year Medical Students. *Annals of Internal Medicine* 114:482–489.
Bredfeldt, Raymond, Jerry A. Colliver, and Robert M. Wesley
   1989   Present Status of Obstetrics in Family Practice and the Effects of Malpractice Issues. *Journal of Family Practice* 28 (3): 294–297.
Brennan, Troyen
   1991   *Just Doctoring: Medical Ethics in the Liberal State.* Berkeley, Los Angeles, Oxford: University of California Press.
Brennan, Troyen, Liesi Hebert, Nan M. Laird, Ann G. Lawthers, Kenneth E. Thorpe, Lucian L. Leape, A. Russell Localio, Stuart R. Lipsitz, Joseph P. Newhouse, Paul C. Weiler, and Howard H. Hiatt
   1991   Hospital Characteristics Associated with Adverse Events and Negligent Care. *Journal of the American Medical Association* 265: 3265.
Brennan, Troyen, Lucian L. Leape, Nan M. Laird, Liesi Hebert, A. Russell Localio, Ann G. Lawthers, Joseph P. Newhouse, Paul C. Weiler, and Howard H. Hiatt
   1991   Incidence of Adverse Events and Negligent Care in Hospitalized Patients. *New England Journal of Medicine* 321:431.
Broder, Samuel
   1994   Fraud in Breast Cancer Trials. Correspondence. *New England Journal of Medicine,* May 19, 1994: 1460–1461.
Brody, Howard, and Kenneth R. Howe
   1987   Maternity Care in Family Practice. Commentary. *Journal of Family Practice* 25 (3): 241–242.
Brooks, Peter
   1984   *Reading for the Plot: Design and Intention in Narrative.* New York: Vintage Books.
Bruner, Jerome
   1986   *Actual Minds, Possible Worlds.* Cambridge, Mass.: Harvard University Press.
   1990   *Acts of Meaning.* Cambridge, Mass.: Harvard University Press.
Campion, Francis X., ed.
   1990   *Grand Rounds on Medical Malpractice.* The Risk Management Foundation of the Harvard Medical Institutions Incorporated. Milwaukee: American Medical Assoc.
Colombotos, John, and Corinne Kirchner
   1986   *Physicians and Social Change.* New York: Oxford University Press.

Colwell, Jack M.
    1992   Where Have All the Primary Care Applicants Gone? *New England Journal of Medicine* 326 (6): 387–393.
Comaroff, Jean
    1982   Medicine: Symbol and Ideology. In *The Problem of Medical Knowledge,* ed. P. Wright and A. Treacher. Edinburgh: Edinburgh University Press.
    1985   *Body of Power, Spirit of Resistance: The Culture and History of a South African People.* Chicago: University of Chicago Press.
Conrad, Peter, and Eugene Gallagher
    1993   *Sociological Perspectives in International Health.* Philadelphia: Temple University Press.
Conrad, Peter, and Rochelle Kern
    1986   *The Sociology of Health and Illness: Critical Perspectives in Medical Sociology.* New York: St. Martin's Press.
Crabtree, B. F., and W. L. Miller
    1991   A Qualitative Approach to Primary Care Research: The Long Interview. *Family Medicine* 23 (2): 145–151.
Crouse, Byron J.
    1989   Family Physicians' Involvement in Obstetric Care: Rural Northeastern Minnesota and Northwestern Wisconsin. *Journal of Family Practice* 28 (6): 724–727.
Davis-Floyd, Robbie
    1992   *Birth as an American Rite of Passage.* Berkeley, Los Angeles, Oxford: University of California Press.
DesMarchais, J.
    1991   Designing a Doctor: From Traditional to Problem-based Curriculum: How the Switch Was Made at Sherbrooke, Canada. *The Lancet* 338 (July 27): 234–237.
Eco, Umberto
    1994   *Six Walks in the Fictional Woods.* Cambridge, Mass.: Harvard University Press.
Eichhorn, John H., et al.
    1990   Standards for Patient Monitoring during Anesthesia at Harvard Medical School. *Journal of the American Medical Association,* August 1986. Reprinted in *Grand Rounds on Medical Malpractice,* ed. F. X. Campion (Milwaukee: American Medical Assoc.).
Eisenberg, Leon
    1992   Sounding Board: Treating Depression and Anxiety in Primary Care: Closing the Gap between Knowledge and Practice. *New England Journal of Medicine* 326:1080–1084.
    1993   It Is Not Morally Acceptable to Require Individual Physicians at the Bedside to Make Cost-Control Rationing Decisions. Lecture delivered at Grossmont Hospital Tenth Annual Symposium on Cancer Care, San Diego, January 30.
Enarson, Cam, and Frederic Burg
    1992   An Overview of Reform Initiatives in Medical Education: 1906–

1992. *Journal of the American Medical Association* 268:1141–1143.

Estroff, Sue
  1981   *Making It Crazy.* Berkeley, Los Angeles, London: University of California Press.
  1989   Self, Identity, and Subjective Experience of Schizophrenia: In Search of the Subject. *Schizophrenia Bulletin* 15:189–196.

Fabian, Johannes
  1971   Language, History, and Anthropology. *Philosophy of the Social Sciences* 1:19–47.

Family Practice, Journal of
  1989 Letters. *Journal of Family Practice,* vol. 29: 361, 443, 604, 606.

Farmer, Paul
  1988   Bad Blood, Spoiled Milk: Bodily Fluids as Moral Barometers in Rural Haiti. *American Ethnologist* 15:62–83.
  1990a   AIDS and Accusation: Haiti, Haitians, and the Geography of Blame. In *Culture and AIDS,* ed. Douglas A. Feldman. New York: Praeger Publishers.
  1990b   Sending Sickness: Sorcery, Politics, and Changing Concepts of AIDS in Rural Haiti. *Medical Anthropology Quarterly* 4:6–27.
  1992   *AIDS and Accusation: Haiti and the Geography of Blame.* Berkeley, Los Angeles, Oxford: University of California Press.

Farmer, Paul, Shirley Lindenbaum, and Mary-Jo DelVecchio Good
  1993   Women, Poverty, and AIDS: An Introduction. *Culture, Medicine, and Psychiatry* 17 (4): 387–397.

Farrow, Diana C., William C. Hunt, and Jonathan M. Samet
  1992   Geographic Variation in the Treatment of Localized Breast Cancer. *New England Journal of Medicine,* vol. 326, no. 17, April 23, 1992: 1097–1101.

Fisher, Bernard, and Carol K. Redmond
  1994   Fraud in Breast Cancer Trials. Correspondence. *New England Journal of Medicine,* May 19, 1994: 1458–1460.

Fisher, Sue, and Alexandra Dundas Todd, eds.
  1983   *The Social Organization of Doctor-Patient Communication.* Washington, D.C.: Center for Applied Linguistics.

Fox, Renee C.
  1959   *Experiment Perilous: Physicians and Patients Facing the Unknown.* Glencoe, Ill.: Free Press.
  1980   The Evolution of Medical Uncertainty. *Milbank Quarterly* 58: 1–49.
  1988   *Essays in Medical Sociology: Journeys into the Field.* 2d ed. New York: John Wiley and Sons.
  1992   *Spare Parts: Organ Replacement in American Society.* With Judith Swazey. New York: Oxford University Press.

Frankenberg, Ronald
  1988a   Gramsci, Marxism, and Phenomenology: Essays for the Development of Critical Medical Anthropology. R. Frankenberg, ed. Special Issue of *Medical Anthropology Quarterly* 2 (4): 324–459.

1988b   Gramsci, Culture, and Medical Anthropology: Kundry and Parsifal? or Rat's Tail to Sea Serpent? *Medical Anthropology Quarterly* 2:324–337.

1988c   "Your Time or Mine?" An Anthropological View of the Tragic Temporal Contradictions of Biomedical Practice. *International Journal of Health Services* 18:11–34.

1993   Risk: Anthropological and Epidemiological Narratives of Prevention. In *Knowledge, Power, and Practice: The Anthropology of Medicine in Everyday Life*, ed. Shirley Lindenbaum and Margaret Lock. Berkeley, Los Angeles, Oxford: University of California Press.

Freidson, Eliot

1970a   *Professional Dominance: The Social Structure of Medical Care.* New York: Atherton Press.

1979b   *The Profession of Medicine: A Study of the Sociology of Applied Knowledge.* New York: Dodd, Mead and Co.

1975   *Doctoring Together: A Study of Professional Social Control.* Chicago: University of Chicago Press.

1986   *Professional Powers: A Study of the Institutionalization of Formal Knowledge.* Chicago: University of Chicago Press.

1989   *Medical Work in America: Essays on Health Care.* New Haven, Conn.: Yale University Press.

Frigoletto, Fredric

1989   Conference Proceedings, transcribed (October 1987). The Medical Malpractice Crisis in Obstetrics, Kenneth Ryan et al. Boston: Harvard University.

Gaines, Atwood D.

1979   Definitions and Diagnoses. *Culture, Medicine and Psychiatry* 3: 381–418.

1982   Cultural Definitions, Behavior, and the Person in American Psychiatry. In *Cultural Conceptions of Mental Health and Illness*, ed. A. Marsella and G. White. Dordrecht: D. Reidel Publishing Co.

1992a   Ethnopsychiatry: The Cultural Construction of Psychiatries. In *Ethnopsychiatry: The Cultural Construction of Folk and Professional Psychiatries*, ed. A. D. Gaines. Albany, N.Y.: State University of New York Press.

1992b   From DSM-I to III-R; Voices of Self, Mastery, and the Other: A Cultural Constructivist Reading of U.S. Psychiatric Classification. *Social Science and Medicine* 35 (1): 3–24.

Gani, Lusia, Herawati Arif, Swa Kurniati Widjaja, Rianto Adi, Heru Prasadja, Lamtiur H. Tampubolon, Eduard Lukito, and Robert Jauri

1991   Physicians' Prescribing Practice for Treatment of Acute Diarrhoea in Young Children in Jakarta. *Journal of Diarrhoeal Diseases Research* 9 (3): 194–199.

Garnick, Hendricks, and Troyen Brennan

1991   Can Practice Guidelines Reduce the Numbers of Malpractice Claims? *Journal of the American Medical Association* 266:2856–2860.

Geertz, Clifford
1965   *A Social History of an Indonesian Town.* Cambridge, Mass.: MIT
        Press.
Geyman, John P.
1989   Toward the Resolution of Generalist-Specialist Boundary Issues.
        Editorial. *Journal of Family Practice* 28 (4): 399–400.
Gifford, Sandra M.
1986   The Meaning of Lumps: A Case Study of the Ambiguities of Risk.
        In *Anthropology and Epidemiology: Interdisciplinary Approaches to
        the Study of Health and Disease,* ed. Craig R. Jones, Ron Stall, and
        Sandra M. Gifford. Dordrecht: D. Reidel Publishing Company.
Good, Byron J.
1994   *Medicine, Rationality, and Experience.* Cambridge, England: Cam-
        bridge University Press.
Good, Byron J., and Mary-Jo DelVecchio Good
1980   The Meaning of Symptoms: A Cultural Hermeneutic Model for
        Clinical Practice. In *The Relevance of Social Science for Medicine,*
        ed. L. Eisenberg and A. Kleinman. Dordrecht: D. Reidel Publish-
        ing Co.
1981   The Semantics of Medical Discourse. In *Sciences and Cultures,*
        Sociology of the Sciences, vol. 5, ed. E. Mendelsohn and Y. El-
        kana. Dordrecht: D. Reidel Publishing Co.
1993   "Learning Medicine": The Constructing of Medical Knowledge
        at Harvard Medical School. In *Knowledge, Power, and Practice:
        The Anthropology of Medicine in Everyday Life,* ed. Shirley Linden-
        baum and Margaret Lock. Berkeley, Los Angeles, Oxford: Uni-
        versity of California Press.
Good, Bryon J., Mary-Jo DelVecchio Good, and Robert Moradi
1985   The Interpretation of Dysphoric Affect and Depressive Illness in
        Iranian Culture. In *Culture and Depression,* ed. Arthur Kleinman
        and Byron Good. Berkeley, Los Angeles, London: University of
        California Press.
Good, Mary-Jo DelVecchio
1985   Discourses on Physician Competence. In *Physicians of Western
        Medicine,* ed. R. Rahn and A. Gaines. Dordrecht: D. Reidel Pub-
        lishing Co.
1990   The Practice of Biomedicine and the Discourse on Hope: A Pre-
        liminary Investigation into the Culture of American Oncology. In
        *Anthropologies of Medicine: A Colloquium on West European and
        North American Perspectives,* ed. Beatrix Pfleiderer and Gilles Bi-
        beau. Heidelberg, Germany: Vieweg.
1994   Medicine on the Edge: Conversations with Oncologists. In *Sci-
        ence, Technology, and Culture,* ed. George Marcus. Chicago: Uni-
        versity of Chicago Press (forthcoming).
Good, Mary-Jo DelVecchio, and Byron J. Good
1989   "Disabling Practitioners": Hazards of Learning to Be a Doctor in
        American Medical Education. *Journal of Orthopsychiatry* 59:303–
        309.

Good, Mary-Jo DelVecchio, Byron Good, and Paul Cleary
1987   Do Patient Attitudes Influence Physician Recognition of Psycho-social Problems in Primary Care? *Journal of Family Practice* 25: 53–59.

Good, Mary-Jo DelVecchio, Byron J. Good, Cynthia Schaffer, and Stuart E. Lind
1990   American Oncology and the Discourse on Hope. *Culture, Medicine, and Psychiatry* 14:59–79.

Good, Mary-Jo DelVecchio, Linda Hunt, Tseunetsugu Munakata, and Yasuki Kobayashi
1993   A Comparative Analysis of the Culture of Biomedicine: Disclosure and Consequences for Treatment in the Practice of Oncology. In *Sociological Perspectives in International Health,* ed. Peter Conrad and Eugene Gallagher. Philadelphia: Temple University Press.

Good, Mary-Jo DelVecchio, Tsunetsugu Munakata, Yasuki Kobayashi, Cheryl Mattingly, and Byron J. Good
1994   Oncology and Narrative Time. *Social Science and Medicine* 38 (6): 855–862.

Gordon, Deborah R.
1988   Tenacious Assumptions in Western Medicine. In *Biomedicine Examined,* ed. Margaret Lock and Deborah Gordon. Dordrecht: Kluwer Academic Publishers.
1990   Embodying Illness, Embodying Cancer. *Culture, Medicine, and Psychiatry* 14:275–297.

Gupta, Geeta Rao, and Ellen Weiss
1993   Women's Lives and Sex: Implications for AIDS Prevention. *Culture, Medicine, and Psychiatry* 17 (4): 399–412.

Haas, J., and W. Shaffir
1991   *Becoming Doctors: The Adoption of a Cloak of Competence.* Greenwich, Conn.: JAO Press.

Hafferty, Frederic W.
1988   Cadaver Stories and the Emotional Socialization of Medical Students. *Health and Social Behavior* 29:344–356.
1991   *Into the Valley: Death and the Socialization of Medical Students.* New Haven, Conn.: Yale University Press.

Hahn, Robert A.
1985   A World of Internal Medicine: Portrait of an Internist. In *Physicians of Western Medicine,* ed. R. A. Hahn and A. D. Gaines. Dordrecht: D. Reidel Publishing Co.
1987a   Patient, Technique, and Voice in American Obstetrics. Guest editorial. *Medical Anthropology Quarterly* 1 (3): 227–229.
1987b   Divisions of Labor: Obstetrician, Woman, and Society in *Williams Obstetrics,* 1903–1985. Special issue, *Medical Anthropology Quarterly* 1 (3): 256–282.

Hahn, Robert A., and Atwood Gaines, ed.
1985   *Physicians of Western Medicine.* Dordrecht: D. Reidel Publishing Co.

Haraway, Donna Jeanne
1993   The Biopolitics of Postmodern Bodies: Determination of Self in
        Immune System Discourse. In *Knowledge, Power, and Practice: The
        Anthropology of Medicine and Everyday Life,* ed. Shirley Linden-
        baum and Margaret Lock, 364–410. Berkeley, Los Angeles, Ox-
        ford: University of California Press.

Harvard Medical Practice Study
1990   Patients, Doctors, and Lawyers: Medical Injury, Malpractice Lit-
        igation, and Patient Compensation in New York. Cambridge,
        Mass.: Harvard University.

Herdt, Gilbert, and Shirley Lindenbaum, eds.
1992   *The Time of AIDS: Social Analysis, Theory, and Method.* London:
        Sage Publications.

Hiatt, Howard
1975   Protecting the Medical Commons: Who Is Responsible? *New En-
        gland Journal of Medicine* 293:235.

Hilfiker, David
1984   Facing Our Mistakes. *New England Journal of Medicine* 310 (2):
        118–122.
1985   *Healing the Wounds: A Physician Looks at His Work.* New York:
        Pantheon Press.

Holland, Jimmie C.
1989   Now We Tell—But How Well? *Journal of Clinical Oncology* 7 (5):
        557–559.

Holland, J. C., N. Geary, A. Marchini, S. Tross
1987   An International Survey of Physician Attitudes and Practice in
        Regard to Revealing the Diagnosis of Cancer. *Cancer Investiga-
        tion* 5:151–154.

Holzer, J. F.
1990a   The Advent of Clinical Standards for Professional Liability. In
        Grand Rounds on Medical Malpractice, ed. F. X. Campion. Mil-
        waukee: American Medical Assoc.
1990b   Current Concepts in Risk Management, 1984. In *Grand Rounds
        on Medical Malpractice,* ed. F. X. Campion. Milwaukee: American
        Medical Assoc.

Huet, P.-Michel
1994   Fraud in Breast Cancer Trials. Correspondence. *New England
        Journal of Medicine,* May 19, 1994: 1462.

Hunt, Linda L. M.
1992   *Living with Cancer in Oaxaca, Mexico: Patient and Physician
        Perspectives in Cultural Context.* Ph.D. thesis, Harvard Univer-
        sity, Cambridge, Mass.

Hunter, Katherine
1991   *Doctors' Stories: The Narrative Structure of Medical Knowledge.*
        Princeton, N.J.: Princeton University Press.

IOM (Institute of Medicine)
1989a   *Medical Professional Liability and the Delivery of Obstetrical
        Care.* Committee to Study Medical Professional Liability and the

Delivery of Obstetrical Care. Vol. 1 and vol. 2 (vol. 2 ed. Victoria Rostow and Roger J. Bulger). Washington, D.C.: National Academy Press.

1989b   Medical Professional Liability and the Delivery of Obstetrical Care. *New England Journal of Medicine* 321 (15): 1057–1060.

Iser, Wolfgang
1978   *The Act of Reading: A Theory of Aesthetic Response.* Baltimore: Johns Hopkins University Press.

Johnson, Thomas M., and Carolyn F. Sargent, eds.
1990   *Medical Anthropology: A Handbook of Theory and Method.* New York: Greenwood Press.

Jonas, Harry S.
1987   The Torch Is Passed. Editorial response to AMA and ACOG Council Report. *Journal of the American Medical Association* 258: 3554–3555.

Jordan, Brigitte
1989   Cosmopolitan Obstetrics: Some Insights from the Training of Traditional Midwives. *Social Science and Medicine* 28 (9): 925–937.

1993   *Birth in Four Cultures: A Cross-Cultural Investigation of Childbirth in Yucatan, Holland, Sweden, and the U.S.* Revised and expanded by Robbie Davis-Floyd. Prospect Heights, Ill.: Waveland Press.

Journal of the National Cancer Institute
1994   NCI Issues Information on Falsified Data in NSABP Trials. *Journal of the National Cancer Institute* 86 (7): 487–489.

Kaufert, Patricia
1988   Menopause as Process or Event: The Creation of Definitions in Biomedicine. In *Biomedicine Examined,* ed. M. Lock and D. Gordon. Dordrecht: Kluwer Academic Publishers.

Kirmayer, Laurence J.
1988   Mind and Body as Metaphors: Hidden Values in Biomedicine. In *Biomedicine Examined,* ed. M. Lock and D. Gordon. Dordrecht: Kluwer Academic Publishers.

Klein, Michael
1990   Influence of Perinatal Asphyxia on Neurologic Outcome: Consequences for Family Practice Accoucheurs. *Canadian Family Physician* 36:1735–1740.

1987   Obstetrics Is Too Important to Be Left to the Obstetricians. *Family Medicine* 19:167–169.

Klein, Michael C., R. J. Gauthier, S. H. Jorgensen, J. M. Robbins, J. Kaczorowski, B. Johnson, M. Corriveau, R. Westreich, K. Waghorn, and M. M. Gelfand
1992   Does Episiotomy Prevent Perineal Trauma and Pelvic Floor Relaxation? *Online Journal of Current Clinical Trials,* doc. no. 10 (6019 words; 65 paragraphs), July 1.

Klein, Michael, J. L. Reynolds, F. Boucher, M. Maius, and E. Rosenberg
1984   Obstetrical Practice and Training in Canadian Family Medicine:

Conserving an Endangered Species. *Canadian Family Physician* 30:2093–2098.

Kleinman, Arthur M.
1980   *Patients and Healers in the Context of Culture: An Exploration of the Borderland between Anthropology, Medicine, and Psychiatry.* Berkeley, Los Angeles, London: University of California Press.
1986   *Social Origins of Distress and Disease: Depression, Neurasthenia, and Pain in Modern China.* New Haven, Conn.: Yale University Press.
1988a   *Rethinking Psychiatry: From Cultural Category to Personal Experience.* New York: Free Press.
1988b   *The Illness Narratives: Suffering, Healing, and the Human Condition.* New York: Basic Books.

Kleinman, Arthur, and Byron J. Good, eds.
1985   *Culture and Depression: Studies in the Anthropology and Cross-Cultural Psychiatry of Affect and Disorder.* Berkeley, Los Angeles, London: University of California Press.

Kolligian, John
1990   Perceived Fraudulence as a Dimension of Perceived Incompetence. In *Competence Considered,* ed. R. Sternberg and J. Kolligian. New Haven, Conn.: Yale University Press.

Kriebel, Stephen H., and James D. Pitts
1988   Obstetric Outcomes in a Rural Family Practice: An Eight-Year Experience. *Journal of Family Practice* 27 (4): 377–384.

Kruse, Jerry, Debra Phillips, and Robert M. Wesley
1989   Factors Influencing Changes in Obstetric Care Provided by Family Physicians: A National Study. (Second article from study.) *Journal of Family Practice* 28 (5): 597–602.

Kuipers, Joe C.
1989   "Medical Discourse" in Anthropological Context: Views of Language and Power. *Medical Anthropology Quarterly* 3:99–123.

Langer, Ellen, and Kwangyang Park
1990   Incompetence: A Conceptual Reconsideration. In *Competence Considered,* ed. R. Sternberg and J. Kolligian. New Haven, Conn.: Yale University Press.

Leape, Lucian, Troyen Brennan, Nan M. Laird, Ann G. Lawthers, A. Russell Localio, Benjamin Barnes, Liesi Hebert, Joseph P. Newhouse, Paul C. Weiler, and Howard H. Hiatt
1991   The Nature of Adverse Events in Hospitalized Patients. *New England Journal of Medicine* 324:377–384.

LeFevre, Michael, Harold L. Williamson, and Melvin Hector
1989   Obstetrics Risk Assessment in Rural Practice. *Journal of Family Practice* 28 (6): 691–696.

Light, Donald
1979   Uncertainty and Control in Professional Training. *Journal of Health and Social Behavior* 20:310–322.
1980   *Becoming Psychiatrists: The Professional Transformation of Self.* New York: W. W. Norton and Co.

1983   Medical and Nursing Education: Surface Behavior and Deep Struc-
         ture. In *Handbook of Health, Health Care, and the Health Profes-
         sions,* ed. David Mechanic. New York: Free Press.
1988   Toward a New Sociology of Medical Education. *Journal of Health
         and Social Behavior* 29:307–322.
Light, Donald, and Sol Levine
1988   The Changing Character of the Medical Profession: A Theoreti-
         cal Overview. *Milbank Quarterly* 66 (2): 10–32.
Lind, Stuart E.
1986   Fee-for-Service Research. *New England Journal of Medicine* 314:
         312–315.
Lind, Stuart E., Mary-Jo D. Good, C. S. Minkovitz, and Byron J. Good
1991   Oncologists Vary in Their Willingness to Undertake Anti-Cancer
         Therapies. *British Journal of Cancer* 64:391–395.
Lind, Stuart E., Mary-Jo D. Good, Steven Seidel, Thomas Csordas, and
Byron J. Good
1989   Telling the Diagnosis of Cancer. *Journal of Clinical Oncology* 7:
         563–589.
Lind, Stuart E., Daniel Kopans, and Mary-Jo DelVecchio Good
1992   Patients' Preferences for Learning the Results of Mammographic
         Examinations. *Breast Cancer Research and Treatment* 23:223–232.
Lindenbaum, Shirley, and Margaret Lock, eds.
1993   *Knowledge, Power, and Practice: The Anthropology of Medicine and
         Everyday Life.* Berkeley, Los Angeles, Oxford: University of Cali-
         fornia Press.
Localio, A. Russell, Ann G. Lawthers, Troyen A. Brennan, Nan M. Laird,
Liese E. Hebert, Lynn M. Peterson, Joseph P. Newhouse, Paul C. Weiler, and
Howard H. Hiatt
1991   Relation between Malpractice Claims and Adverse Events due to
         Negligence: Findings from the Harvard Medical Practice Study,
         III. *New England Journal of Medicine* 325:245–251.
Lock, Margaret
1988   Introduction. In *Biomedicine Examined,* ed. Margaret Lock and
         Deborah Gordon. Dordrecht: Kluwer Academic Publishers.
1990   On Being Ethnic: The Politics of Identity Breaking and Making
         in Canada, or, *Nevra* on Sunday. *Culture, Medicine, and Psychi-
         atry* 14:237–254.
Lock, Margaret, and Deborah Gordon, eds.
1988   *Biomedicine Examined.* Dordrecht: Kluwer Academic Publishers.
Lock, Margaret, and Nancy Scheper-Hughes
1990   A Critical-Interpretive Approach in Medical Anthropology: Rit-
         uals and Routines of Discipline and Dissent. In *Medical Anthro-
         pology: A Handbook of Theory and Method,* ed. T. Johnson and
         C. Sargent. New York: Greenwood Press.
Lomas, Jonathan, Geoffrey M. Anderson, Karin Domick-Pierre, Walter J.
Hannah, and Eugene Vayda
1989   Do Practice Guidelines Guide Practice?: The Effect of a Con-

sensus Statement on the Practice of Physicians. *New England Journal of Medicine* 321:1306–1311.

Love, Susan M.
1991   *Dr. Susan Love's Breast Book.* Reading, Mass.: Addison-Wesley Publishing Co.

Ludmerer, Kenneth
1985   *Learning to Heal: The Development of American Medical Education.* New York: Basic Books.

Maretzki, Thomas W.
1985   Biomedicine and Naturopathic Healing in West Germany: A Historical Ethnomedical View of a Stormy Relationship. *Culture, Medicine, and Psychiatry* 9:383–422.

1989   Cultural Variation in Biomedicine: The *Kur* in West Germany. *Medical Anthropology Quarterly* 3:22–35.

Marston, Robert Q.
1992   Robert Wood Johnson Foundation Commission on Medical Education: The Sciences of Medical Practice, Summary Report. *Journal of the American Medical Association* 268:1144–1145.

Marston, Robert Q., and Roseann M. Jones, eds.
1992   *Medical Education in Transition: Commission on Medical Education: The Sciences of Medical Practice.* Princeton, N.J.: Robert Wood Johnson Foundation.

Martin, Emily
1987   *The Woman in the Body: A Cultural Analysis of Reproduction.* Boston: Beacon Press.

1993   Histories of Immune Systems. *Culture, Medicine, and Psychiatry* 17 (1): 67–76.

Martini, Carlos J. M.
1988   Evaluating the Competence of Health Professionals. *Journal of the American Medical Association* 260 (8): 1057–1058.

Mattingly, Cheryl
1989   Thinking with Stories: Story and Experience in a Clinical Practice. Ph.D. thesis, Massachusetts Institute of Technology, Cambridge, Mass.

1991   The Narrative Nature of Clinical Reasoning. *Journal of American Occupational Therapy* 45:998–1005.

1994   The Concept of Therapeutic "Emplotment." *Social Science and Medicine* 38 (6): 811–822.

Mattingly, Cheryl, and Linda C. Garro
1994   Introduction. *Social Science and Medicine* 38 (6): 771–774.

McKinlay, John B.
1986   A Case for Refocusing Upstream: The Political Economy of Illness. In *The Sociology of Health and Illness: Critical Perspectives,* ed. P. Conrad and R. Kern. New York: St. Martin's Press.

1988   Introduction: The Changing Character of the Medical Profession. *Milbank Quarterly* 66 (2): 1–9.

Mechanic, David
1992   Some Thoughts about the Behavioral and Social Sciences and

Medical Education. In *Medical Education in Transition,* ed. R. Q. Marston and R. M. Jones. Princeton, N.J.: Robert Wood Johnson Foundation.

1994   *Inescapable Decisions: The Imperatives of Health Reform.* New Brunswick, N.J.: Transaction Publishers.

Mechanic, David, ed.

1983   *Handbook of Health, Health Care, and the Health Professions.* New York: Free Press.

Mengel, Mark B., and William R. Phillips

1987   The Quality of OB Care in Family Practice: Are Family Physicians as Safe as Obstetricians? *Journal of Family Practice* 24 (2): 159–164.

Merton, Robert K., G. G. Reader, and P. L. Kendall

1957   *The Student-Physician: Introductory Studies in the Sociology of Medical Education.* Cambridge, Mass.: Harvard University Press for the Commonwealth Fund.

Milbank Quarterly

1988   Special Issue, "The Changing Character of the Medical Profession," vol. 66, supplement 2.

Millman, Marcia

1977   *The Unkindest Cut: Life in the Backrooms of Medicine.* New York: William Morrow and Co.

Minnesota Medical Insurance Exchange

1988   OB Risk Management Guidelines Approved: Risk Management Review. *Minnesota Medicine* 71:567–568.

Mishler, Elliot

1986a   *The Discourse of Medicine: Dialectics of Medical Interviews.* Norwood, N.J.: ABLEX.

1986b   *Research Interviewing: Context and Narrative.* Cambridge, Mass.: Harvard University Press.

Mizrahi, Terry

1986   *Getting Rid of Patients: Contradictions in the Socialization of Physicians.* New Brunswick, N.J.: Rutgers University Press.

Moore, Gordon T.

1992   The Case of the Disappearing Generalist: Does It Need to Be Solved? *Milbank Quarterly* 70 (2): 361–379.

Moore, Gordon T., Susan D. Block, and Regina Mitchell

1990   A Randomized Controlled Trial Evaluating the Impact of the New Pathway Curriculum at Harvard Medical School. Report to the Fund for the Improvement of Post-Secondary Education.

1994   An Evaluation of the Impact of the New Pathway Curriculum on Harvard Medical Students. *Academic Medicine,* forthcoming, fall.

Moore, Sally Falk

1987   Explaining the Present: Theoretical Dilemmas in Processual Ethnography. *American Ethnologist* 14:727–736.

Morgan, John

1765   *A Discourse upon the Institution of Medical Schools in America.*

Philadelphia: William Bradford. Quoted in *The Student Physician,* by Robert Merton, G. G. Reader, and P. L. Kendall (Cambridge, Mass.: Harvard University Press for the Commonwealth Fund, 1957).

Morgan, Lynn M.
1990   The Medicalization of Anthropology: A Critical Perspective on the Critical-Clinical Debate. *Social Science and Medicine* 30:945–950.

Morsy, Soheir
1990   Political Economy in Medical Anthropology. In *Medical Anthropology: A Handbook of Theory and Method,* ed. Thomas M. Johnson and Carolyn F. Sargent. New York: Greenwood Press.

Mulkay, Michael
1981   Action and Belief or Scientific Discourse? *Philosophy of the Social Sciences* 11:163–171.

Mulkay, Michael, and G. N. Gilbert
1982a   Joking Apart: Some Recommendations Concerning the Analysis of Scientific Culture. *Social Studies of Science* 12:585–613.
1982b   Warranting Scientific Belief. *Social Studies of Science* 12:383–408.

Mulkay, Michael, J. Potter, and S. Yearly
1983   Why an Analysis of Scientific Discourse Is Needed. In *Science Observed: Perspectives on the Social Study of Science,* ed. K. Knorr-Cettina and M. Mulkay. Beverly Hills, Calif.: Sage Publications.

Nattinger, Ann Butler, Mark S. Gottlieb, Judith Veum, David Yahnke, and James S. Goodwin
1992   Geographic Variation in the Use of Breast-Conserving Treatment for Breast Cancer. *New England Journal of Medicine,* vol. 326, no. 17 (April 23): 1102–1107.

Navarro, Vicente
1988   Professional Dominance or Proletarianization? Neither. *Milbank Quarterly* 66 (2): 57–75.

Nelson, Karin
1988   What Proportion of Cerebral Palsy Is Related to Birth Asphyxia? *Journal of Pediatrics* 112:572–573.

Nelson, Karin H., and J. H. Ellenberg
1984   Obstetric Complications as Risk Factors for Cerebral Palsy or Seizure Disorders. *Journal of the American Medical Association* 251: 1843–1848.
1986   Antecedents of Cerebral Palsy: Multivariate Analysis of Risk. *New England Journal of Medicine* 315:81–86.

Novack, Dennis H., Robin Plumer, Raymond L. Smith, Herbert Ochitill, Gary R. Morrow, and John M. Bennett
1979   Changes in Physicians' Attitudes toward Telling the Cancer Patient. *Journal of the American Medical Association* 241:897–903.

Office of Educational Development, Harvard Medical School
1989   The New Pathway to General Medical Education at Harvard University. *Teaching and Learning in Medicine* 1:42–46.

Oken, Donald
    1961   What to Tell Cancer Patients: A Study of Medical Attitudes. *Journal of the American Medical Association* 175:1120–1128.
Oldham, Robert K.
    1987   Sounding Board: Patient-Funded Cancer Research. *New England Journal of Medicine* 316:46–47.
O'Neil, Edward H.
    1992   Education as Part of the Health Care Solution: Strategies from the Pew Health Professions Commission. *Journal of the American Medical Association* 268:1146–1148.
Ong, Aihwa
    1987   *Spirits of Resistance and Capitalist Discipline: Factory Women in Malaysia.* Albany, N.Y.: State University of New York Press.
    1988   The Production of Possession: Spirits and the Multinational Corporation in Malaysia. *American Ethnologist* 15:28–42.
Onion, Daniel K., and Anne M. Mockapetris
    1988   Specialty Bias in Obstetric Care for High Risk Socioeconomic Groups in Maine. *Journal of Family Practice* 27 (4): 423–427.
Ornstein, Steven M., Mindy A. Smith, James Peggs, David Garr, and June Gonzales
    1990   Obstetric Ultrasound by Family Physicians: Adequacy as Assessed by Pregnancy Outcome. *Journal of Family Practice* 30 (4): 403–408.
Ortiz, Ana
    1994   Healers in the Storm: Dominican Health Practitioners Confront the Debt Crisis. Ph.D. dissertation (draft), Harvard University, Cambridge, Mass.
Paci, Eugenio
    1993   Culture and Biomedicine: The Case of Oncology. Presentation to Medical Anthropology Seminar, Harvard University, October 22.
Paget, Mary Ann
    1982   Your Son Is Cured Now: You May Take Him Home. In *Physicians of Western Medicine: Five Cultural Studies,* Special Issue, ed. Atwood T. Gaines and Robert A. Hahn. *Culture, Medicine, and Psychiatry* 6 (3): 237–259.
    1988   *The Unity of Mistakes: A Phenomenological Interpretation of Medical Work.* Philadelphia: Temple University Press.
Parsons, Talcott
    1978   The Sick Role and the Role of the Physician Reconsidered. In *Action Theory and the Human Condition.* New York: Free Press.
Petersdorf, Robert
    1983   Sounding Board: Is the Establishment Defensible? *New England Journal of Medicine* 309:1053–1087.
    1986   Medical Schools and Research: Is the Tail Wagging the Dog? *Daedalus* 115:99–118.
    1992   Primary Care Applicants—They Get No Respect. *New England Journal of Medicine* 326 (6): 408–409.

Peterson, Lynn, and Troyen Brennan
   1990   Medical Ethics and Medical Injuries: Taking Our Duties Seriously. *Journal of Clinical Ethics* 1 (3): 207–211.
Peterson, Thomas C., Paul J. Reiss, and William C. Wadland
   1990   Restructuring a Family Practice Obstetrics Curriculum. *Journal of Family Practice* 30 (1): 81–85.
Pivnick, Anitra
   1993   HIV Infection and the Meaning of Condoms. *Culture, Medicine, and Psychiatry* 17 (4): 431–453.
Poisson, Roger
   1994   Fraud in Breast Cancer Trials. Correspondence. *New England Journal of Medicine,* May 19, 1994: 1460.
Primary Care Task Force (AMA)
   1992   Report of the Medical Schools Section Primary Care Task Force. *Journal of the American Medical Association* 268:1092–1094.
Rabinow, Paul
   1993   Galton's Regret and DNA Typing. *Culture, Medicine, and Psychiatry* 17 (1): 59–65.
Rakel, Robert E.
   1989   Family Practice: Journal of the American Medical Association Review of Specialties. *Journal of the American Medical Association* 261 (19): 2845–2846.
Relman, Arnold
   1980   The New Medical-Industrial Complex. *New England Journal of Medicine* 303:963–970.
   1989   Medical Professional Liability and the Relations between Doctors and Their Patients. In *Medical Professional Liability and the Delivery of Obstetrical Care.* Vol. 2: *Institute of Medicine,* ed. V. Rostow and R. Bulger. Washington, D.C.: National Academy Press.
   1990   Changing the Malpractice Liability System. *New England Journal of Medicine* 322 (9): 626–627.
   1992   "Self Referral"—What's at Stake? *New England Journal of Medicine* 327:1522–1524.
Rennie, Drummond
   1994   Breast Cancer: How to Mishandle Misconduct. *Journal of the American Medical Association* 271 (15): 1205–1207.
Rhodes, Lorna Amarasingham
   1990   Studying Biomedicine as a Cultural System. In *Medical Anthropology: A Handbook of Theory and Method,* ed. T. Johnson and C. Sargent. New York: Greenwood Press.
   1991   *Emptying Beds: The Work of an Emergency Psychiatric Unit.* Berkeley, Los Angeles, Oxford: University of California Press.
Richer, Gilles
   1994   Fraud in Breast Cancer Trials. Correspondence. *New England Journal of Medicine,* May 19, 1994: 1462.
Ricoeur, Paul
   1981a   *Hermeneutics and the Human Sciences.* Edited and translated by John B. Thompson. Cambridge, England: Cambridge University Press.

1981b   Narrative Time. In *On Narrative,* ed. W. J. T. Mitchell. Chicago:
University of Chicago Press.

1984   *Time and Narrative.* Vol. I. Translated by Kathleen McLaughlin
and David Pellauer. Chicago: University of Chicago Press.

Roback, Gene, Lillian Randolph, and Bradley Seidman

1992   *Physician Characteristics and Distribution in the U.S.* Milwaukee:
American Medical Assoc.

Roberts, Marc J., with Alexandra T. Clyde

1993   *Your Money or Your Life: The Health Care Crisis Explained.* New
York: Doubleday.

Robertson, William O.

1988   Access to Obstetric Care: A Growing Crisis. Guest editorial. *Journal of Family Practice* 27 (4): 361–362.

Rooks, Judith P., Norman L. Weathersby, Eunice K. M. Ernst, Susan Sta-
pleton, David Rosen, and Allan Rosenfield

1989   Outcomes of Care in Birth Centers. *New England Journal of Medicine* 321 (26): 1804–1808.

Rosenblatt, Roger A.

1988   The Future of Obstetrics in Family Practice: Time for a New Direction. *Journal of Family Practice* 26:127–129.

Ryan, Kenneth J. (and Conference Participants)

1989   The Medical Malpractice Crisis in Obstetrics: The Economic, Medical, and Health Policy Implications. Transcription of proceedings
of conference held at Harvard University, October 10, 1987.
Boston: Division of Health Policy Research and Education, Harvard University. (Kenneth J. Ryan, M.D., Chair of the Department of Obstetrics, Gynecology, and Reproductive Biology, was
conference chairman.) Participants included Julius B. Richmond,
M.D., and Don Harper Mills, M.D., J.D., as ex-officio members,
and physicians, lawyers, and insurance and policy specialists who
made up the medical, insurance, and legal panels. Individual comments from the conference proceedings are quoted under the
name of participant. The proceedings are referenced as Ryan et al.
1989.

Savage, Wendy

1986   *A Savage Enquiry: Who Controls Childbirth?* London: Virago.

Sayres, William G.

1989   Letter: Obstetric Risk Assessment. *Journal of Family Practice* 28
(3): 266, 328–329.

Scheper-Hughes, Nancy

1990   Three Propositions for a Critically Applied Medical Anthropology. *Social Science and Medicine* 30:189–197.

Scheper-Hughes, Nancy, and Margaret M. Lock

1987   The Mindful Body: A Prolegomenon to Future Work in Medical
Anthropology. *Medical Anthropology Quarterly* 1:6–41.

Scherger, Joseph E.

1987   The Family Physician Delivering Babies: An Endangered Species.
Family Medicine 19 (2): 95–96.

1988   Assessing Obstetric Risk: Commentary. *Journal of Family Practice* 27:162–163.

Scherger, Joseph, and Jeffrey Tanji
1988   Family Physicians Strive to Continue Obstetrics. *California Family Physician* 38:12–13.

Schiller, Nina Glick
1993   The Invisible Women: Caregiving and the Construction of AIDS Health Services. *Culture, Medicine, and Psychiatry* 17 (4): 487–512.

Schmittling, Gordon, and Carole Tsou
1989   Obstetric Privileges for Family Physicians: A National Study. *Journal of Family Practice* 29 (2): 179–184.

Schwartz, William, and Daniel N. Mendelson
1989   Physicians Who Have Lost Their Malpractice Insurance. *Journal of the American Medical Association.* 262 (10): 1335.

Scott, James
1985   *Weapons of the Weak: Everyday Forms of Peasant Resistance.* New Haven, Conn.: Yale University Press.

1990   *Domination and the Arts of Resistance: Hidden Transcripts.* New Haven, Conn.: Yale University Press.

Shy, Kirkwood K., David A. Luthy, Forrest C. Bennett, Michael Whitfield, Eric B. Larson, Gerald van Belle, James P. Hughes, Judith A. Wilson, and Morton A. Stenchever
1990   Effects of Electronic Fetal-Heart-Rate Monitoring, as Compared with Periodic Auscultation, on the Neurologic Development of Premature Infants. *New England Journal of Medicine* 322 (9): 588–593.

Smith, Mindy A., Lee A. Green, and Thomas L. Schwenk
1989   Family Practice Obstetrics in Michigan: Factors Affecting Physician Participation. *Journal of Family Practice* 28 (4): 433–437.

Smucker, Douglas R.
1988   Obstetrics in Family Practice in the State of Ohio. *Journal of Family Practice* 26 (2): 165–168.

Sobo, E. J.
1993   Inner-City Women and AIDS: The Psycho-Social Benefits of Unsafe Sex. *Culture, Medicine, and Psychiatry* 17 (4): 455–485.

Starr, Paul
1982   *The Social Transformation of American Medicine.* New York: Basic Books.

Sternberg, Robert, and John Kolligian, eds.
1990   *Competence Considered.* New Haven, Conn.: Yale University Press.

Stewart, William L.
1989   Obstetrics in Family Practice. Letter to the Editor. *Journal of Family Practice* 29 (6): 606.

Stoeckle, John
1988   Reflections on Modern Doctoring. *Milbank Quarterly* 66 (2): 76–91.

Stossel, Thomas
    1987   Brave New Medicine: Presidential Address to the American So-
            ciety of Clinical Investigation, San Diego, May 2.
Swinbanks, David
    1989a   Japanese Doctors Keep Quiet. *Nature* 339:409.
    1989b   Cancer Drugs Restrictions Recommended. *Nature* 339:843.
Taylor, Kathryn M.
    1988   Physicians and Disclosure of Undesirable Information. In *Biomed-
            icine Examined,* ed. Margaret Lock and Deborah Gordon. Dor-
            drecht: Kluwer Academic Publishers.
Tietze, Paul E., Samuel E. Gaskins, and Mary Joyce McGinnis
    1988   Attrition from Obstetrical Practice among Family Practice Resi-
            dency Graduates. *Journal of Family Practice* 26 (2): 204–205.
Todd, Alexandra
    1989   *Intimate Adversaries: Cultural Conflict between Doctors and Women
            Patients.* Philadelphia: University of Pennsylvania Press.
Todd, James S.
    1990   Publisher's Commentary. In *Grand Rounds on Medical Malprac-
            tice,* ed. Francis X. Campion. Milwaukee: American Medical Assoc.
Todorov, Tzvetan
    1984   *Mikhail Bakhtin: The Dialogical Principle.* Translated by Wlad
            Godzich. Minneapolis: University of Minnesota Press.
Tosteson, Daniel C.
    1981   Science, Medicine, and Education. The Alan Gregg Memorial
            Lecture. *Journal of Medical Education* 56:8–15.
Traweek, Sharon
    1993   An Introduction to Cultural and Social Studies of Science and
            Technologies. *Culture, Medicine, and Psychiatry* 17 (1): 3–25.
Treichler, Paula A.
    1992   AIDS, HIV, and the Cultural Construction of Reality. In *The
            Time of AIDS: Social Analysis, Theory, and Method,* ed. Gilbert
            Herdt and Shirley Lindenbaum. London: Sage Publications.
Waitzkin, Howard
    1981   The Social Origins of Illness: A Neglected History. *International
            Journal of Health Services* 11:77–103.
    1991   *The Politics of Medical Encounters: How Patients and Doctors Deal
            with Social Problems.* New Haven, Conn.: Yale University Press.
Wall, Eric M.
    1988   Assessing Obstetric Risk: A Review of the Obstetric Risk-Scoring
            Systems. *Journal of Family Practice* 27 (2): 153–163.
Wall, Eric M., Ann E. Sinclair, Jared Nelson, and William L. Toffler
    1989   The Relationship between Assessed Obstetric Risk and Maternal-
            Perinatal Outcome. *Journal of Family Practice* 28 (1): 35–40.
Ward, Martha C.
    1993   A Different Disease: HIV/AIDS and Health Care for Women in
            Poverty. *Culture, Medicine, and Psychiatry* 17 (4): 413–430.

Weiler, Paul C.
   1991   *Medical Malpractice on Trial.* Cambridge, Mass.: Harvard University Press.
Weiler, Paul C., Howard H. Hiatt, Joseph P. Newhouse, William G. Johnson, Troyen A. Brennan, and Lucian L. Leape
   1993   *A Measure of Malpractice: Medical Injury, Malpractice Litigation, and Patient Compensation.* Cambridge, Mass.: Harvard University Press.
Weinstein, Michael M.
   1994   The Freedom to Choose Doctors: What Freedom? *New York Times Magazine,* March 27.
West, Candace
   1984   *Routine Complications: Troubles with Talks between Doctors and Patients.* Bloomington: Indiana University Press.
Westbrook, Lisa, and Dorian M. Patchin
   1988   Malpractice and Obstetrics. *Business and Health* 5 (May 1988): 56.
White, Hayden
   1976   The Fictions of Factual Representation. In *The Literature of Fact,* ed. A. Fletcher. New York: Columbia University Press.
   1981   The Value of Narrativity in the Representation of Reality. In *On Narrative,* ed. W. J. T. Mitchell. Chicago: University of Chicago Press.
William, L.
   1989   The Relationship between Assessed Obstetric Risk and Maternal-Perinatal Outcome. *Journal of Family Practice* 28 (1): 35–40.
Williams, Albert P., William B. Schwartz, Joseph P. Newhouse, and Bruce W. Bennett
   1983   How Many Miles to the Doctor? *New England Journal of Medicine* 309:958–963.
Young, Allan
   1981   The Creation of Medical Knowledge: Some Problems in Interpretation. *Social Science and Medicine* 15B:379–386.
   1990   Moral Conflicts in a Psychiatric Hospital Treating Combat-Related Posttraumatic Stress Disorder (PTSD). In *Social Science Perspectives on Medical Ethics,* ed. George Weisz. Dordrecht: Kluwer Academic Publishers.

Index

Designer: U.C. Press Staff
Compositor: Prestige Typography
Text: 10/13 Galliard
Display: Galliard
Printer: Thomson-Shore, Inc.
Binder: Thomson-Shore, Inc.